MAGICAL MILES

2016 EDITION

The Runner's Guide to

Walt Disney World®

All information in this guidebook is subject to change. We recommend that you call ahead to obtain current information before traveling.

Please consult with your doctor before starting any exercise regimen.

ISBN 978-0-9884443-6-2

Printed in the United States of America.

Table of Contents

Acknowledgements

Every runner can use some crowd support to motivate them to cross the finish line. We would like to thank those who have helped us run this race! To Kristina Murphy, Kim Bruch, and Nicole Amare, Associate Professor at University of South Alabama, for reviewing our initial manuscript; to Seventy7 Designs who did a fantastic job creating our cover design; to Marc D. Baldwin, PhD, Owner & CEO of Edit911; to our Sanborn's team: Mark Johnstone, President of Sanborn's Travel Service, for his leadership and Jenna Sampson, Operations Manager of Sanborn's Travel Service, for all her help in making things run smoothly; to Cara Goldsbury, Chief Executive Concierge of Glass Slipper Concierge, for your editing, inspiration, support, and mentoring; to Bill Downs, Disney Destinations District Sales Manager for your direction and support; and finally to our husbands, Scot Albrecht and Brent Biller, who have not only dealt with our craziness throughout the writing process, but have been extremely supportive of our book. Thank you for allowing us to follow our dreams!

Megan's Dedication

To my parents, who brought me up in a loving, Christian home, while instilling the concept of hard work into my life. The legacy passed down from my grandparents and through you both is proof of hard work and family values. You are, and always will be, my role models. I love you both!

To my wonderful husband, who truly is my best friend. He has supported me throughout my running journey and even tags along as my personal photographer and cheerleader. I cannot thank God enough for placing the perfect man in my life, to stand beside me as we continue on our journey together!

To my brother, who never ceases to remind me that I am not, in fact, perfect. I remind him that I am, however, older and wiser. Even though you may tease me, you push me to be a better person, and I love you for it.

Most importantly, to God for blessing me with wonderful family, and this amazing opportunity.

And to Krista. I am so blessed to have such an incredible co-author, but most importantly amazing friend in you!

Krista's Dedication

As a young adult, I had never been particularly athletic and I had never even considered being a runner. In fact, as a young child, I wore braces on my legs. It was only through the Jeff Galloway Run/Walk/Run method that I was able to complete my first distance race, the NYC Marathon. Since that first race, I've used the Galloway Method to train and complete every race I've ran. And, while I've never met Jeff Galloway (nor is this a paid endorsement) I would like to thank him for inspiring athletes from the average to the elite. I can truly say that without Jeff, not only would I have never crossed a finish line but chances are I would never have crossed a starting line.

To my parents and aunts, thank you for inspiring me to be my best. Especially to my aunt, Jean Cooper, who at an early age taught me to believe that anything was possible through hard work.

To my loving husband, Scot who (even though he is much faster) will run along side me at any race when I ask. If he runs at his own pace, he always returns to cross the finish line with me. I am so happy to have you to run the race of life with every day!

To my beautiful daughter, Addison whose laugh can light up any room. I am so honored to be your mother. It is because of you that I strive to be a better person every day.

To God, who has blessed me with amazing people in my life!

And, to Megan. Not only was it a true joy to have God place you in my life as a fantastic co-author but also a friend!

Foreword

Over the last 50 years, I have attended over 1000 events, giving advice, hearing from runners and watching how runners relate to one another. The runDisney events have a special positive energy and cooperative atmosphere. No other series has introduced running to more people with a blend of experiences for veterans. You can expect to "run happy" at a runDisney event.

My wife Barbara and I look forward to every runDisney event. There is a high quality of organization, with interesting entertainment. The festive atmosphere inspires a high percentage of the participants to dress up and become part of the fun.

At every event I meet a steady stream of family groups, pulling one another into fitness. Thousands of these "newbies" have openly admitted that they would not have agreed to this family challenge at a non-Disney venue.

Amazing are the life-changing stories in which unhealthy people become fit because they wanted to win their medal at WDW or Disneyland. Then they saw the next series of medals...and the Coast to Coast emblem. They were hooked!

I'm often asked "which event is the best?". My response is simple and heartfelt: "They are like children—each is different". Each has a special atmosphere that pulls even hardcore runners into the theme. There is no other organization that can consistently provide such creative musical and visual effects. If there were a world record for smiles, it would be set at the runDisney finish line.

At a recent runDisney expo, I asked a veteran participant why she kept coming back. Her response says it all: I have a lot of challenges in my life. When I go to a runDisney event I get all of benefits to mind and spirit and I'm happy the whole weekend."

Enjoy this comprehensive guide and I look forward to seeing you during race weekend.

Jeff Galloway
US Olympian
Official Training Consultant
runDisney

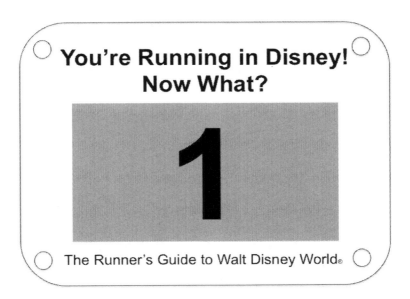

You're Running in Disney! Now What?

1

The Runner's Guide to Walt Disney World®

More popular than ever, runDisney races are selling out faster than in previous years. This year alone, we've seen an increase in the number of events offered. As we embarked on the second edition of the *Runner's Guide to Walt Disney World*, our goal was and is to give detailed information on how to make your race weekend a stress-free racecation.

What's New in 2016?

In the fourth edition of the *Runner's Guide to Walt Disney World*, we've added a chapter that includes the history of runDisney as well as what goes into planning these massive race weekends. Jeff Galloway has also added a special message in the training chapter. The newest runDisney race weekends, including the Star Wars Half-Marathon Weekend – The Dark Side, have been added to this most recent edition. runDisney has continued to make changes to enhance the runner experience, so we have included information on those changes as well. To add further dimension to our book, we've continued to incorporate reader reviews and comments on many of the popular events and attractions associated with Walt Disney World and runDisney.

What makes runDisney events unique?

In 2014, the Walt Disney World Marathon was given the number 7 spot in the largest marathons in the nation (and finished in the thirteenth spot in the world)[i]. Disney races also took three spots in the top fifteen half-marathons in the nation and two spots in the top fifteen half-marathons in the world[ii]. In 2014 alone, Disney hosted over 200,000 participants in their events.

If you are even considering running a race at Disney, know that you're one of many with a taste for a fun challenge. Around half of runDisney event participants are new runners experiencing their first race or have never participated in a runDisney event before. You are in great company as you get ready to tighten up your running shoes and experience Disney in a fun and unique way.

If you have ever visited a Disney park, you know the excitement of meeting various Disney characters. Now imagine your excitement when you meet them while running a race. Disney continues to spread its magic by offering great character meet-and-greet opportunities along each course. You may even see a few rare characters that do not regularly appear at the theme parks throughout Walt Disney World.

At runDisney events, the excitement goes beyond just the characters. Even celebrities participate in the runDisney excitement. Don't be surprised to see some of your favorite TV personalities at a runDisney event, especially Walt Disney World Marathon Weekend.

[i] *Running USA.* (2014). Retrieved September 2015, from http://www.runningusa.org/marathon-report-2015?returnTo=annual-reports

[ii] *Running USA.* (2014). Retrieved September 2015, from http://www.runningusa.org/half-marathon-report-2015?returnTo=annual-reports

One thing that makes a runDisney event truly special is that there is something for everyone. From the longer distances or multi-day challenges for the adults, the 5K for every member of your family, and the Kids' Races for the little ones, everyone will be able to participate in these amazing events. For those who would rather watch, there are many great opportunities to cheer on your runner. And where else can you end your race with a magical family vacation?

How Will This Book Help?

You can use this book to help select a race that is best for you, but there are so many more aspects of your racecation to consider. This book will discuss the many resort options, including the proximity to the parks and race courses. We will also discuss ticket types, dining plans, and food. Yes, even the restaurant descriptions are provided with a runner's diet in mind. After all, you need to fuel your body properly the night before and have a great celebration meal after you've completed your race.

It's no secret that runners enjoy having friends and family along the course to support them through their race. Inside are tips for the spectators to make sure they are able not only to watch you along the course, but also enjoy the entertainment of the race while they cheer you on.

Let's admit it, while at Walt Disney World, you'll want to experience the parks, right? There is an entire section devoted to navigating the parks with ease, especially the day prior to your race. Those legs will want to be well rested before your big event.

Perhaps you have run a small race in your hometown and you are ready to branch out to longer distances. This race could be your first or your fiftieth. What makes Disney different? Disney knows efficiency and how to entertain. From stepping off the plane to getting back to your resort after the race, all aspects of the event run like a well-oiled machine. With amazing volunteers, fun entertainment, and great sponsors, Disney races are like no other. And don't forget the medal! Disney is known for creating amazing medals for their events, something that keeps runners coming back for more.

There are people of all shapes, sizes, ethnicities, and genders that participate in these events. There are first-time runners, and there are veteran runners. There are those participating in their first runDisney event and those who keep coming back. However, you are all there for the same reasons: to stay healthy and active, to have fun, and to smile as you run through a Disney park.

What makes it even more special is that Disney celebrates every runner. Everyone who crosses the finish line is given the same amount of excitement and hoopla. You may be the first, the last, or somewhere in the middle, but you are encouraged and celebrated as you complete what you have trained to do.

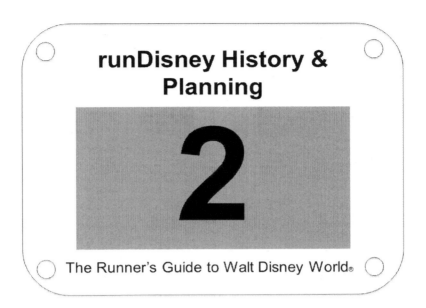

runDisney History & Planning

2

The Runner's Guide to Walt Disney World®

Races have been occurring on Walt Disney World property since 1994. Formerly called the Disney Endurance Series, events included races like the original Walt Disney World Marathon and other races not produced by Disney.

As the interest in running increased, Disney decided to change the name and begin to add to the race events. With the allure of running through the Disney theme parks and the unique medals, the draw for the events was undoubtedly increasing. In 2010, runDisney emerged and soon many more race weekends were added to the mix.

runDisney not only expanded their race portfolio, new race distances were also included. Series of events, including shorter distances, proved to be a big hit. To make it a truly family-friendly event, Kids' Races were also included. As the race weekends continued to grow, the themes emerged including new franchises like Star Wars and Marvel, appealing to another new crowd of runners.

runDisney Race History

1994 – First Annual Walt Disney World Marathon

1998 – Fifth Annual Walt Disney World Marathon includes Disney's Wide World of Sports Complex in its 26.2-mile course for the first time. 13,000 runners ran up and back Victory Way between mile markers 19 and 20. This is the first year that a half-marathon event is also included.

2003 – Walt Disney World Marathon and Half-Marathon celebrates its 10th annual event with a record 22,000 registered participants (16,000 in the full marathon), including 149 "Perfect 10 Club" runners who competed in their 10th Walt Disney World Marathon event.

2004 – Inaugural Florida Half Ironman Triathlon at Walt Disney World Resort features a 1.2-mile swim, a 56-mile bike and a 13.1-mile run and serves as a qualifier for the Ironman World Championship in Kona, Hawaii. A total of 1,970 athletes competed in the event.

2005 – The Walt Disney World Triathlon occurs for the first time with approximately 1,000 competitors racing through a 1.5K swim, 40K bike ride, and a 10K run that starts at Disney's Contemporary Resort and ends at Epcot.

2006 – The Inaugural Disney's Minnie Marathon Weekend kicks off an innovative new women's sports initiative. More than 2,000 athletes participated in the Go Red for Women 5K, one mile fun run/walk or the Women Run the Work 15K.

2006 – Disneyland Half-Marathon marks the first endurance series on the west coast. More than 9,700 runners participated in the inaugural half-marathon, an event affectionately dubbed "The Happiest Race on Earth".

2006 – More than 1,500 tri-athletes participated in the Walt Disney World Triathlon, making it the largest field in event history.

2008 – The first annual Expedition Everest Challenge took place at Disney's Animal Kingdom. The event was a nighttime 5K race that progressed into an obstacle course and a scavenger hunt for the runners as they made their way through the theme park.

2009 – The inaugural Disney Princess Half-Marathon Weekend was held at Walt Disney World. More than 11,000 runners competed in various races throughout the weekend, making this event one of the largest endurance race weekends geared towards women.

2009 – The final Tower of Terror 13K race was held at Disney's Hollywood Studios.

2010 – The new runDisney brand was announced, bringing together all four current Disney marathon and half-marathon weekends to create a unique series of destination races that offer one-of-a-kind running experiences.

2010 – A sold out field of runners (11,000) experienced the inaugural Wine & Dine Half-Marathon Weekend at Walt Disney World Resort. The half-marathon was the first runDisney event held at night and the first to involve a relay option.

2012 – The inaugural Tinker Bell Half-Marathon at Disneyland Resort led runners on a 13.1-mile trek through the parks, as well as several city of Anaheim landmarks. Over 12,000 registered runners took part in this event.

2012 – A record 27,000 athletes took part in a variety of Disney's Princess Half-Marathon Weekend events, with a field of 19,000 for the half-marathon event alone.

2012 – The scarily popular Twilight Zone Tower of Terror themed runDisney race returned in the form of an inaugural 10-miler weekend at Disney's Hollywood Studios.

2014 – The 21st annual Walt Disney World Marathon Weekend became the first 5-day race weekend in runDisney history. This year featured the inaugural WDW 10K and the inaugural Dopey Challenge.

2014 – More than 15,000 runners competed in the final Twilight Zone Tower of Terror 10-Miler, which was run from Hollywood Studios to ESPN Wide World of Sports Complex and back.

2014 – The inaugural Avengers Super Heroes Half-Marathon Weekend was held at Disneyland Resort. The weekend races included over 17,000 runners from 11 different countries.

2015 – Castaway Cay 5K Challenge was added to the Walt Disney World Marathon Weekend, including over 700 runners.

2015 – More than 23,000 runners participated in the inaugural Star Wars Half-Marathon Weekend at Disneyland Resort.

Race Planning

Ever wonder what goes into planning a runDisney race weekend? First, runDisney personnel begin to brainstorm ideas. In true Disney fashion, an intriguing story is always at the forefront. Whether it be a new franchise, a great movie or even one of the favorite characters, a race weekend revolves around this story. And if enough guests speak up, one of your favorite extinct races may even make a reappearance!

The next 18 months are devoted to making the race weekend's story come to life. Discussions property-wide begin, primarily with Operations and Reedy Creek. The main areas of discussion revolve around how the race weekend will impact the property. How will road closures affect traffic? Will guests not participating in the race be impacted? Will there be any construction in the parks? Once everything is addressed, a date can be made and the course planning can begin.

When it comes to course design, there is much to consider. Along with road closures, overall distance (all distances are USTAF certified), construction, and the like, guest experience is also considered. Although course crowding does occur, runDisney does their best to make sure the course will accommodate the race field size. Another consideration is the amount of time the race will take (with the pace limit) to open up the roads and parks to all guests.

From there, it's a matter of preparing the property and cast members for the upcoming event! Thousands of people are involved in making sure the race weekend is a magical experience for all.

In terms of recurring events, the planning time may not be as long, however it is still just as extensive. After each race weekend, the team meets to determine if any changes need to be made. If it is a big change, such as dates or location, the process is similar to putting together a new race. Otherwise, the runDisney crew looks at the logistics and guest experience to determine if any smaller changes, such as race capacity or slight course adjustments, need to be made.

Registration for the races usually goes on sale 9 months before the race weekend. This not only allows for the runDisney team to prepare for the event, but also for the runners to properly train and make travel arrangements. From there, the planning continues including race day logistics, shirt and medal designs, expo planning and much more.

Race Numbers

While the number of race weekends and runners has definitely increased since 2010, the overall numbers for each weekend has remained quite consistent in the past year or two. This is primarily due to the fact that every race weekend sells out! In 2014, runDisney hosted over 200,000 runners in Walt Disney World.

The Health & Fitness Expo brings in the largest numbers during a race weekend. When you include the guests of runners and locals, over 1.5 times the number of registered runners attend the expo. This is a prime location for vendors and with a space as large as the ESPN Wide World of Sports Complex, many can join in on the fun.

After a race weekend, the runDisney team will meet to discuss guest experience on the course. If there was quite a bit of course crowding, the race capacity may be smaller the next year. If they are able to adjust the course, it may mean a slightly larger race capacity. However, the overall numbers tend to remain the same.

runDisney races continue to be a draw for the beginning runners and each race showcases just that. Over half of registered runners state that it is their first runDisney race or even their first race in general! Most of the other registered runners are those who experience the magic of the races and bring their friends to keep coming back for more.

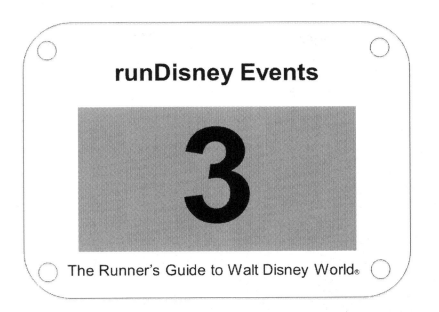

runDisney Events

The Runner's Guide to Walt Disney World®

There are currently nine runDisney events held throughout the year, with four events in Disneyland, four events in Walt Disney World and beginning in 2016, an event in Disneyland Paris. In 2015, an extension of one event was added to the Disney Cruise Line as well. The largest is the Walt Disney World Marathon Weekend with over 50,000 runners. The Princess Half-Marathon and Tinker Bell Half-Marathon have a higher demographic of women participants but men are more than welcome to register and run. Each event offers opportunities for kids as well as fun activities before and after the main events.

Walt Disney World Marathon Weekend - January

There is no better way to start off the new year than participating in the largest runDisney event. Held around the second weekend in January, this event brings in the most participants because there are multiple races.

Starting with the Health and Fitness Expo, you can get hands-on exposure to multiple vendors related to running and fitness. Try out new shoes, get samples of running fuel, and much more. It's located at the ESPN Wide World of Sports Complex, and transportation is provided from every Disney resort at Walt Disney World. There are four days to enjoy the Walt Disney World Marathon Weekend Expo: Wednesday, Thursday, Friday, and Saturday. The Expo usually opens mid-morning and stays open until late afternoon.

The kids can also get in on the fun by participating in their own races. Anyone thirteen or under can participate. There is even a diaper division. Allow your children the opportunity to run on the track and show their athletic prowess while vacationing at Walt Disney World. All kids participating in the races receive a medal. These races are located on the field at ESPN Wide World of Sports behind the expo location.

The Kids' Races are held on Thursday, Friday, and Saturday of the race weekend. The Kids' Dashes are late morning, followed by the Mickey Mile each day. Be sure to allow enough time to get from a main race to ESPN Wide World of Sports for the Kids' Races.

As every runner knows, you need to eat your carbs before a big event. Disney knows too. Experience the Pasta in the Park Party, held in Epcot three different nights throughout the weekend. Enjoy a pasta buffet dinner while a DJ keeps you entertained. There are even appearances from your favorite Disney characters. Be sure to stay until the end to enjoy your private viewing location for Epcot's laser and firework show, Illuminations: Reflections of Earth. Pasta in the Park starts at 7:00 p.m. on Thursday, Friday, and Saturday.

The weekend's main events are the Family Fun Run 5K (3.1 miles) on Thursday morning, Walt Disney World 10K (6.2 miles) on Friday morning, Walt Disney World Half-Marathon (13.1 miles) on Saturday morning, Walt Disney World Marathon (26.2 miles) on Sunday morning, and the increasingly popular Goofy's Race-and-a-Half Challenge, which is a 39.3-mile challenge for runners participating in both the half-marathon and marathon. For the truly crazy is the Dopey Challenge, which includes the 5K, 10K, half-marathon, and marathon races, 48.6 miles of fun.

The Family Fun Run 5K begins at 6:00 a.m. Thursday. Enjoy running (or walking) through Epcot while meeting up with your favorite Disney characters. Runners ages five and older are encouraged to participate. (The stroller divisions have been removed.)

The Walt Disney World 10K begins at 5:30 a.m. on Friday morning. The course takes you through Epcot and around the Epcot resorts.

Starting at 5:30 a.m. on Saturday, the Walt Disney World Half-Marathon includes 13.1 miles of magic as the course takes you through Magic Kingdom and Epcot.

On Sunday, the Walt Disney World Marathon begins at 5:30 a.m. and includes 26.2 miles throughout the Walt Disney World Resort, including all four theme parks as well as ESPN Wide World of Sports Complex.

For those brave (or goofy) enough to participate in both the half-marathon and marathon, then Goofy's Race-and-a-Half Challenge is just for you. Race in both Saturday and Sunday morning events and receive *three* medals in the end.

If you want an even greater challenge, participate in the 5K, 10K, half-marathon, and marathon races and receive a whopping *six* medals by completing the Dopey Challenge!

A great way to end the weekend is with an after party in Disney Springs on Sunday evening. After all that running, you deserve to have some fun. From 2-8 p.m., head to the Westside with your friends and family for some dancing, music, food, and more. Admission is free and open to the public.

Castaway Cay Challenge – January

Who wouldn't love to add a Disney Cruise to their Walt Disney World Marathon Weekend fun? In 2015, the addition of the Castaway Cay Challenge was created.

Participate in one of the races during the Walt Disney World Marathon Weekend (5K or longer), then set sail for 4-nights in the Bahamas on the Disney Dream the Monday after race weekend. During your stop at Castaway Cay, participate in an early morning Castaway Cay 5K. Along with your finisher's medallion, you will receive an extra Castaway Cay Challenge medal.

Along with the race challenge, there will be many special activities onboard including healthy menu options, exclusive merchandise and even runDisney-related fun.

Star Wars Half-Marathon Weekend - January

Is the force strong with you? Occurring in mid-January (one week after Walt Disney World Marathon Weekend) at Disneyland Resort, this is sure to be a popular race weekend.

The weekend begins with the Health and Fitness Expo. Here you can explore the various vendors, showcasing the best in running and fitness. You can also experience the speaker series, which includes talks from Jeff Galloway, Tara Gidus, race directors and more. It is located at the Disneyland Hotel and is open on Thursday, Friday and Saturday.

On Friday morning, the Star Wars 5K will take place. This is a family-friendly 3.1 mile event that is sure to include a lot of great entertainment as you run through the Disneyland Resort.

The Star Wars 10K will held on Saturday morning. This 6.2 mile course will take you through Disneyland and California Adventure parks.

Even the tiniest Padawans can join in on the fun! The Star Wars Kids Races will occur on Saturday at 10:00 a.m. From diaper dashers to 8 year olds, there is a fun race for everyone.

The main event, the Star Wars Half-Marathon, is on Sunday morning. This 13.1 mile journey will take you through Disneyland and California Adventure parks, as well as along the streets of Anaheim.

For those wanting the ultimate Jedi test, take on the 10K and half-marathon races as part of the Rebel Challenge. Along with the individual 10K and half-marathon medals, receive a special Rebel Challenge medal as well.

Princess Half-Marathon Weekend - February

Cinderella had a glass running shoe. Call up your girlfriends and enjoy a weekend of princess fun. You may even bring (or meet) your Prince Charming as men can participate too.

Start off with the Fit for a Princess Expo, where you will arrive on a red carpet. Shop to your heart's content with various vendors, many catering specifically to women. The expo is located at the ESPN Wide World of Sports Complex, and there is transportation available from the Disney host resorts. The expo is open on Thursday, Friday, and Saturday from mid-morning to late afternoon.

For those wanting to make their weekend even more special, be sure to experience the Pasta in the Park Party at Epcot. Enjoy a pasta buffet and stay to watch Illuminations: Reflections of Earth from a special viewing location. The party begins at 7:00 p.m. on Friday and Saturday.

On Friday morning, lace up your running shoes for the Royal Family 5K. This is a family-friendly 3.1-mile run through Epcot. Take photos with your favorite Disney characters, and be sure to smile.

After the Royal Family 5K, stay and enjoy the Princess Half-Marathon Breakfast. Located in the family reunion area in Epcot, this breakfast occurs on Friday and Saturday mornings from 6:30-8:30 a.m.

Enchanted 10K race will be held on Saturday morning.

Allow your little princess and prince to experience the weekend by participating in the Kids' Races. On Friday and Saturday mornings at Epcot, kids thirteen and younger can run their own race and even get a medal.

The weekend concludes with the main event, the Princess Half-Marathon. On Sunday at 5:30 a.m., women (and a few charming men) lace up their slippers for a 13.1-mile trek.

For those wanting the royal treatment, participate in the 10K and Half-Marathon races as part of the Glass Slipper Challenge. Along with the individual 10K and half-marathon medals, receive a special Glass Slipper Challenge medal as well.

Once the running is over, head to Disney Springs for the Happily Ever After Party. From 2-8 p.m., enjoy delicious food, great music and even grab another keepsake or two. Admission is free and is open to the public.

Star Wars Half-Marathon – The Dark Side – April

Join the dark side at Walt Disney World during the inaugural Star Wars Half-Marathon Weekend. With the success of this race on the west coast, it has been brought to the east coast by popular demand in 2016.

Begin your galactic journey with the Health and Fitness Expo. Located at ESPN Wide World of Sports, runners can get their hands on the latest running gear and listen to speakers. The expo will be held on Thursday, Friday and Saturday.

On Friday, the Star Wars 5K begins at Epcot. This 3.1 mile adventure is for the entire family.

The Star Wars 10K looks to be a new course, beginning at Epcot and ending at ESPN Wide World of Sports. The race begins on Saturday and includes a 6.2 mile trek along with visits from your favorite characters.

Saturday also includes the Kids' Races. Located at the ESPN Wide World of Sports Complex, the littlest of Padawans can see if they can escape the dark side.

On Sunday, the Star Wars Half-Marathon takes place. The course appears to begin in Epcot and end at ESPN Wide World of Sports Complex. See if the force is strong with you during this 13.1 mile journey.

For those wanting to spend more time with the dark side, take on the Dark Side Challenge by completing the Star Wars 10K and Star Wars Half Marathon and receive another medal.

Tinker Bell Half-Marathon - May

You can fly. Test out your faith, trust, and pixie dust in this 13.1-mile race through Disneyland and the surrounding areas of Anaheim.

The weekend begins with the Health and Fitness Expo. Once you arrive, you can walk (or take the Anaheim Transportation Network) from any area hotel to the expo located in the Disneyland Hotel. Walk around and visit the vendors, taking in the latest in sports and nutrition. The expo is available on Thursday, Friday and Saturday from mid-morning to late afternoon.

Get the entire family together for the Never Land Family Fun Run 5K. Starting at 5:00 a.m. on Friday, walk, run or fly 3.1 miles through the Disneyland parks. The race begins at the Disneyland Resort.

Spread your wings for the Tinker Bell 10K, starting at 5:30 a.m. on Saturday. This 6.2 mile course will take you throughout Disneyland Resort.

Kids of all ages can participate in the Kids' Races, located in the Disney Springs district. These races are on Saturday morning, following the 10K.

The main event, The Tinker Bell Half-Marathon, begins at 5:30 a.m. on Sunday. Put on your wings, grab your pixie dust, and embark on 13.1 miles through the Disneyland Resort, Disney's California Adventure, and even areas of local Anaheim.

For those wanting to experience a little extra magic, participate in the 10K and Half-Marathon races as part of the Pixie Dust Challenge. Along with the individual 10K and half-marathon medals, receive a special Pixie Dust Challenge medal as well.

Disneyland Half-Marathon - August/September

Get away during Labor Day Weekend and run 13.1 miles through Disneyland Resort, California Adventure, and even through the Anaheim Angels Stadium.

The weekend begins with the Disneyland Health and Fitness Expo. Visit your favorite brands, listen to special speakers, and shop until you drop. It's located at the Disneyland Hotel Exhibit Hall on Thursday, Friday and Saturday from mid-morning to late afternoon.

On Friday beginning at 5:30 a.m., get the entire family together for the Disneyland Family Fun Run 5K. Starting at the Disneyland Resort, enjoy 3.1 miles through the parks.

The Disneyland 10K will begin at 5:30 a.m. on Saturday. This 6.2 mile course will take you throughout the Disneyland Resort, enjoying entertainment along the way.

In Disney Springs, following 10K race, the Kids' Races showcase the athletic talent of the smallest diaper-dasher to the faster kids. Starting at 9 a.m., cheer on your little runner.

For those wanting to carb up before the half-marathon, be sure to experience Pasta in the Park on Saturday evening in Disneyland park. From 6-7:30 p.m., enjoy pasta, salads, and more with other runners and their families.

On Sunday, run 13.1 miles through the original Happiest Place on Earth. The race begins at 5:30 a.m. and winds through Disneyland Resort, Disney's California Adventure, and the city of Anaheim.

For those wanting a greater challenge, participate in both the 10K and Half-Marathon races as part of the Dumbo Double Dare. Along with the individual 10K and half-marathon medals, you will receive a third medal.

Disneyland Paris Half-Marathon Weekend – September

Beginning in 2016, runDisney is going international! The inaugural Disneyland Paris Half-Marathon Weekend opens the gateway into Disney parks across the globe.

This Parisian adventure begins with the Health & Fitness Expo. On Thursday, Friday and Saturday runners can get their race packet and shop from various health-related vendors. The expo is located at the Disney Events Arena.

On Saturday, participants can enjoy the Disneyland Paris 5K. Starting at 7 a.m., this course will take you through Disneyland Paris Park and is a great event for beginners, veterans and families.

Also on Saturday, the youngest of runners can enjoy the Kids' Races. Events include 100 m, 200 m, 400 m, 1K and 2K races and begin at 10 a.m.

Sunday morning is the premier event – the Disneyland Paris Half-Marathon. Starting at 7 a.m., the course will take runners through Walt Disney Studios Park, Disneyland Park and through the countryside and villages.

Wine & Dine Half-Marathon Weekend - November

Do you love the International Food and Wine Festival? Then this event is for you. Enjoy a weekend of food, wine, and running.

Start with the Health and Fitness Expo at the Wide World of Sports where you can talk with representatives of your favorite brands and vendors while finding new ways to enhance your running experience. Transportation is provided from Disney host resorts. The expo is available on Friday and Saturday from mid-morning to late afternoon.

On Saturday at 7 a.m., run Mickey's Jingle Jungle 5K through Animal Kingdom. See your favorite Disney characters along the route as you experience the park in a whole new way.

Kids can participate in their own races on Saturday morning as well. From dashes to a one-mile run, those thirteen and younger can run and receive their own medals. It's located at the ESPN Wide World of Sports Complex beginning at 10 a.m.

Saturday evening, participate in the Wine & Dine Half-Marathon. This race starts at 10 p.m. at ESPN Wide World of Sports.

After the half-marathon, enjoy an after party at Epcot. Ride your favorite attractions, sample international food and wine, and party until 4 a.m. You even get a $15 gift card to use as you like. The party starts at 10:00 p.m.

Avengers Super Heroes Half-Marathon Weekend – November

Let out your inner super hero during this event. Located at Disneyland, this race weekend is sure to be of epic proportions. It is held in mid-November, one week after Wine & Dine Half Marathon Weekend.

Begin your super hero weekend with the Health & Fitness Expo, located in the Disneyland Hotel. Held on Thursday, Friday and Saturday, visit your favorite brands and vendors, as well as enjoy photo opportunities and various speakers.

Even the strongest super heroes need to fuel up. On Friday from 7-8:30 p.m., the Pasta in the Park Party will occur in Disneyland park. Enjoy a pasta buffet, take photos with your favorite super heroes and even experience a few attractions.

Runners of all ages can experience the Super Heroes 5K, starting at 5:30 a.m. on Friday. This 3.1 mile course will take you throughout the Disneyland Resort.

New in 2015 is the Captain America 10K. This race begins at 5:30 a.m. on Saturday and will take you throughout Disneyland Park and Disney's California Adventure.

Even the littlest of super heroes can enjoy the fun. The Kids Races will begin at 9:00 a.m. on Saturday in the Disney Springs District. From diaper dashers to 8 year olds, there is a race for everyone.

Are you ready to test your super powers? The Avengers Super Heroes Half-Marathon is on Sunday at 5:30 a.m. This 13.1 mile course will take you throughout Disneyland and California Adventure parks, as well as along the streets of Anaheim.

For the truly super heroes, take on the Infinity Gauntlet Challenge – new in 2015! This includes the Captain America 10K and Avengers Super Heroes Half-Marathon, resulting in another medal.

Race Extras

For each race weekend, there are usually several race extras associated with each event such as Pasta in the Park, post-race parties, Race Retreat, and ChEAR Squad. (See Chapters 11 and 12.) Separate tickets are required for all events with the exception of the Cool-Down Party (WDW Marathon and Princess Half-Marathon weekends). These events do tend to sell out, so purchase your tickets in advance of your race date.

Coast to Coast Race Challenge

Did you know there is the opportunity for another runDisney medal? All you need to do is complete two Disney races (half-marathon or marathon distances) in both Walt Disney World and Disneyland in the same calendar year and get the Coast to Coast medal. Those who complete the Coast to Coast Challenge will receive their medal upon completion of the second race.

A pink Coast to Coast medal is also offered. For those who run the Princess Half-Marathon and the Tinker Bell Half-Marathon in the same calendar year, you will be awarded a special Coast to Coast medal with a pink overlay and a pink and purple ribbon.

New in 2016 is the Kessel Run Challenge. Complete the Star Wars Half-Marathon in Disneyland followed by the Star Wars Half-Marathon in Walt Disney World in the same calendar year and receive a special medal inspired by the Millennium Falcon starship.

Also beginning in 2016, you can use the same race for multiple Coast to Coast Challenges (including the Coast to Chateau Challenge below). For example, participate in the 2016 Star Wars Half-Marathon in Disneyland in January, along with the 2016 Princess Half-Marathon in Walt Disney World in February, you will receive the classic Coast to Coast medal. If you then participate in the 2016 Tinker Bell Half-Marathon in Disneyland in May, you will also receive the pink Coast to Coast medal.

Castle to Chateau Challenge

For those wanting to take their runDisney experience international, a new challenge is available for 2016! Complete a half-marathon distance at Disneyland Paris, along with a half-marathon distance or longer at Disneyland in California or Walt Disney World in Florida, and you will receive the new Castle to Chateau Challenge medal. These races must occur in the same calendar year.

Anniversary Years

Every five years, each race celebrates its anniversary. What's the big deal with anniversary years? A special medal is created for the race that year. Sometimes even more surprises emerge. (See appendix for inaugural dates to determine when anniversary years are.)

Legacy Runners

Each race has an inaugural year. Participants line up to run the first event of its kind. And then some participants choose to run it again the next year. And the next year. And the next year. Some runners have participated every single year since its first showing. These runners are known as the Legacy Runners for the event. Along with getting their names in the race information packet, they receive a special ribbon on their medal. Be sure to give these runners a high-five as they are truly an inspiration.

In 2013, there were ninety-five Walt Disney World Marathon legacy runners. These runners have completed all twenty Walt Disney World marathons!

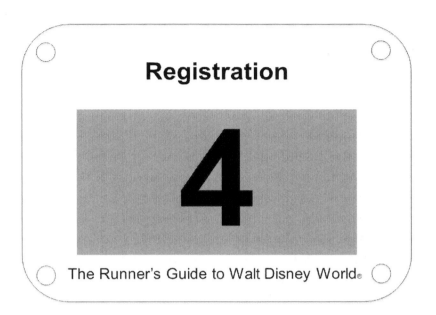

Registration

4

The Runner's Guide to Walt Disney World®

Over the past year, registration for runDisney events has become quite an adventure in itself! Previous years of being able to wait weeks or months after registration open to plan your vacation and register for your race seems to be a thing of the past where runDisney is concerned. With increasing popularity, many of the new runDisney challenges and several races have sold out within days (if not hours) of registration opening to the public. Top the demand for registration with multiple runDisney events throughout the year, and it may be difficult to decide which event to opt for. Here are some considerations to help you choose your magical event and how to register.

Choosing Your Race

There are many things to consider. First, how far do you want to run? With many mileage options ranging from 3.1 miles to 26.2, along with back-to-back challenges, you will need to think about how much training you are able to put into your race preparation, your fitness level, and how long you have to train.

Next, look at the time of year the races occur. When would be the best time to take your kids out of school? What type of weather do you want to train in, and run in? January, February, and November races *usually* mean cooler Florida weather, whereas the April races may be more humid.

Another consideration is deciding if you want to run a morning or night race. Keep in mind that the morning races can start as early as 5:30 a.m. and the night race starts at 10 p.m. The morning races allow you to enjoy the parks in the afternoon. The night race will include an after-party, which is a fun way to celebrate your achievement until the early morning hours.

You may also want to consider the size of the races. Marathon Weekend in January is by far the largest runDisney event. However, with the increasing popularity of runDisney races, most of the key events have between 10,000 and 25,000 runners.

These questions should help you figure out what race is the best for you. And remember, you can always sign up for more than one.

Below is a chart that includes general information about each race. Be sure to check out chapters 14 and 15 for more details about the race courses.

Race	Distance	Month	Start	Course	Finish
WDW 5K	3.1 miles	January	Epcot	Epcot	Epcot
WDW 10K	6.2 miles	January	Epcot	Epcot & Epcot Resorts	Epcot
WDW Half-Marathon	13.1 miles	January	Epcot	Magic Kingdom & Epcot	Epcot
WDW Marathon	26.2 miles	January	Epcot	All 4 theme parks & ESPN	Epcot
Princess 5K	3.1 miles	February	Epcot	Epcot	Epcot
Princess 10K	6.2 miles	February	Epcot	Epcot & Epcot Resorts	Epcot
Princess Half-Marathon	13.1 miles	February	Epcot	Magic Kingdom & Epcot	Epcot
Star Wars 5K	3.1 miles	April	Epcot	Epcot	Epcot
Star Wars 10K	6.2 miles	April	Epcot	TBD	ESPN Complex
Star Wars Half-Marathon	13.1 miles	April	Epcot	TBD	ESPN Complex
Jingle Jungle 5K	3.1 miles	November	Animal Kingdom	Animal Kingdom	Animal Kingdom
Wine & Dine Half-Marathon	13.1 miles	November	ESPN Compex	Animal Kingdom, Hollywood Studios & Epcot	Epcot

Where, When, and How to Register

As the popularity of runDisney events grows, the races have been selling out faster and faster. With the addition of the new challenges, some races and challenges have sold out in a matter of hours. Be

sure to watch the runDisney website or
RunnersGuideToWDW.com for information on registration opening
dates and capacity percentages.

If your race is not yet open for registration, keep an eye on the
runDisney website and sign up for an email reminder to be notified
when registration opens. The email reminders are usually located
on the registration page for each race. In the past, early registration
has been offered for Annual Passholders and Disney Vacation Club
members approximately one or two weeks prior to public
registration. (Note: Early registration is no longer available for
Disney Visa Reward cardholders.) This varies by race, so check the
individual websites for more information. If you have the option of
early registration through one of the above perks, then definitely
take advantage of the option, especially for new races or
challenges, which tend to sell out quickly. Registration always opens
at noon EST.

Once you have chosen which race you are going to participate, your
next step is to head to the runDisney website, **RunDisney.com**.
Click on the race you would like to register for, and then click
REGISTER. Registration for runDisney events is handled through
Active.com, so you will be redirected to their website. Because of
this, it is highly recommended you create an Active.com account
prior to the beginning day of race registration. If you are registering
yourself or children ages 17 and under, use your Active.com
account. If you are registering someone else, you will need to get
their Active.com account information.

There have been instances where the website crashes due to the
amount of activity, so look to runDisney's social media accounts for
new registration website links if this occurs.

Make sure that you pay attention to the prices to take advantage of
discounts due to registering early. To monitor the registration
capacity, keep an eye on the runDisney website. Race capacity will
start to show up on the runDisney website once registrations have
reached 50% for the race. Be careful! Races have been known to

go from 78% full to sold out overnight. Once your race starts to reach 75%, it's time to start seriously thinking about registration.

The sooner you can register, the better. In the past runDisney has provided the option of signing up for future races at the expo of the runDisney race you are attending, but space is very limited and this is becoming much more rare.

When you register, the website will ask you a series of questions. Beyond the normal name, address, and phone number, there will be questions regarding the race. For the 5K and 10K races, you will need to give your estimated pace. Various paces are given for you to choose from. Be honest. You do not want to be trampled by the faster runners, and you do not want to be weaving through the walkers. This is for the safety of all participants. Keep in mind that you must keep at least a sixteen-minute mile pace otherwise you will be swept, or picked up, from the race course without finishing.

For races of half-marathon distance or longer, you will be asked to submit a proof of time through runDisney's website at a later date. This is an official race result of a 10K, 12K, 15K, Half-Marathon or Marathon race in order to be placed into a corral. (For the Walt Disney World Marathon, Goofy's Race-and-a-Half Challenge and Dopey Challenge, you will need to submit a race result of a 10 Mile, Half Marathon or Marathon race.) This proof of time includes the race name, race date, city of the race, race finish time and link to the race results. If you do not submit an official time, you will be placed in the last corral. This proof of time can be submitted up until approximately two months before the race weekend, so make sure you pay close attention to when this needs to be received by. You can no longer bring a proof of time to the Runner Relations booth at the Health and Fitness Expo. See the Proof of Time section below for more information.

Submitting an official race result for corral placement is absolutely vital. Not only does this ensure you will not be put in the last corral, it also places you in a corral with runners of similar pace. If runDisney cannot verify your proof of time through the race result link you provide, you will be placed in the last corral. You can go back to the proof of time link and enter your information to ensure the race result you provided is still accurate.

If you are running with a child, please keep the following age limits in mind: five years and up for 5Ks, ten years and up for 10Ks, fourteen years and up for any of Disney's half-marathon races and the Glass Slipper Challenge, eighteen years and up for the marathon, Goofy's Race-and-a-Half Challenge, and Dopey Challenge.

If you will be participating in the Coast-to-Coast Race Challenge (a race of at least one half-marathon at Disneyland and at least one half-marathon or marathon at Walt Disney World in the same calendar year), you will be automatically entered in this challenge when you register and complete the required combination of races. When you pick up your race packet for the second race of the coast-to-coast challenge, you will be identified as an eligible participant.

For active-duty military, be sure to check the military division. This will not only allow you to earn an award, it may even get you some extra special attention along the way. There are five options for the Army, Navy, Marines, Air Force, or Coast Guard.

If you are a runner with a disability, be sure to indicate that during registration. There is a wheelchair division for runDisney events. For those participating in this event, be sure to mark the appropriate box during registration.

If you have questions, please fill out the contact form on the RunDisney website or call runDisney at 407-938-3398. You have the option of running with a guide, and you can also decide whether you would like to start at the front or within a corral.

Want to sign up for multiple races? For most races, you must sign up for each race individually. The exceptions are the official challenges, such as Goofy's Race-and-a-Half Challenge, the Dopey Challenge, Glass Slipper Challenge, and the Dark Side Challenge.

Since these challenges include multiple events, registering for any challenge will automatically register you in all the races of the challenge.

There are also some commemorative items that you can get during registration. These include pins, commemorative Mickey ears, necklaces, jackets, etc. Keep in mind that these are items you cannot purchase at the expos. If you are interested in purchasing these items, then please definitely put it on your registration form! You pay for these items at time of registration. Usually there are no photos ahead of time, you will find out what they look like when you pick them up at the expo.

Other events to consider when registering are Race Retreat, ChEAR Squad, and Kids' Races, as well as special events such as Pasta in the Park and after parties. For more information on these events, see Chapters 11 and 12.

Do note that there is **no refund** on race registrations and they cannot be transferred to another runner. RunDisney may allow a deferral of registration to the next year for a fee, as is explained later in this chapter.

Your race registration includes a commemorative tech shirt (the Kids' Races and 5K race includes a cotton tee), virtual iGift bag, and race bib. Once you have registered, you will be emailed pre-race briefings, preparing you for the weekend's events along with your race, as well as a post-race email, which includes a link to your personal webpage. This webpage includes your results, your placement among the other runners, multimedia from the event, and a certificate you can download to showcase your accomplishment.

Most races will offer both unisex and a women's cut shirt. The women's shirts do tend to run small, but a size chart for shirts is located on the runDisney website. The shirts are Champion brand.

It is also important to note that there are no waiting lists for runDisney events. Once the race is sold out, it is sold out. If you are at all interested in running a specific race, please register early.

Runner's World Challenge

During the Walt Disney World Marathon Weekend there is a special opportunity for those interested in running the Dopey Challenge, which is the *Runner's World* Challenge. *Runner's World* is one of the premiere running magazines, focusing on all aspects of running. They offer the *Runner's World* Challenge at various races throughout the United States.

The *Runner's World* Challenge package includes your race registration and many other perks and benefits, including a 16-week training plan designed by *Runner's World* experts; a four-month premium membership to a *Runner's World* personal trainer; a *Runner's World* Challenge tech shirt and book; one year of access to the Runner's World Challenge experts on nutrition, injury prevention, and motivation; weekly emails from Chief Running Officer Bart Yasso; private packet pick-up at the Health and Fitness Expo; pre-race course strategy session with *Runner's World* experts; Pasta in the Park Party admission; entry to Race Retreat; preferred corral placement; and an exclusive pre-race walkout to the corrals.

For those interested in registering for the *Runner's World* Challenge, be sure to watch the runDisney and *Runner's World* websites. The registration date may be different from general runDisney registration and sells out quickly. Also, the cost is quite a bit higher than race registration, and the full amount is due at time of registration.

(Note: After the 2016 Walt Disney World Marathon Weekend, there will be a name change to Runner's World VIP.)

Running with a Charity or Team

There are many great opportunities not only to train for a runDisney event, but also to raise money for a charity at the same time. The runDisney website lists the official charity groups for each race. By choosing to register with an official charity group, you are guaranteed a registration for the race, even if the race sells out. There are also specially priced rooms, tickets, and other race events.

You can also run with a local charity group, if you wish. The special benefits above may not apply, but you can make a difference by raising money for a charity, a local nonprofit or one that you personally support.

If a race is sold out, you may be able to get a race registration by partnering with a charity. Check the runDisney website for more information. Be sure to talk with the charity about what is involved so you know up front how much money you need to raise, if you need to get a hotel room with them, and any other information you may need.

Proof of Time

Proof of time is required in order to be placed in a corral other than the last corral. For the half marathon races (or 10K and half marathon challenges), a 10K, 12K, 15K, 10 Mile, Half-Marathon or Marathon race or longer is needed for your proof of time. For the marathon (or Goofy and Dopey Challenges), a 10 Mile, Half-Marathon or Marathon distance race is needed for your proof of time. The proof of time must be within the past 1.5 years. If your proof of time is from a previous runDisney event, you still need to enter your information.

Proof of time must be submitted prior to the deadline for your runDisney event. These deadlines usually occur two months prior to the event. Check the runDisney website or **RunnersGuideToWDW.com** for these deadlines. Be sure to mark down the deadline for submitting your proof of time. This deadline is strict, so if you do not submit your proof of time by this deadline, you will be placed in the last corral.

When looking for a race to get your new proof of time, make sure that it has a certified course. In general, the shorter distances (i.e. 10K for a half marathon or 10 Mile for the marathon) allow you to obtain a faster proof of time. While a destination race is always fun, there are great local races as well.

Once you have your proof of time, go to the runDisney website and click on the race weekend you will be participating in. Under the "Runner Info" tab, scroll to the Proof of Time section. There is a link in which you will include information about your race. Be sure to have the following: name of race, distance, city, state, date and finish time. There also will be a spot to include a link to the race results, ensuring that the race was valid as well as your participation in it. It is recommended that you take a screen shot of your submission and print it for your records.

It cannot be stressed enough that corral placement is for the overall safety of all participants. Be honest when submitting your estimated finish time and race proof of time. If your race result cannot be verified, you will be placed in the last corral. You can return to the proof of time link before the deadline to ensure your proof of time submission is still accurate. If you have any questions, contact runDisney or Track Shack.

Volunteering

Whether you are local or traveling to cheer on your runner, you have the opportunity to participate in a runDisney event in a distinct way by volunteering. Each race requires lots of hands to make sure that everything runs smoothly. From the expo to the race itself, volunteers (or sports enthusiasts) are welcomed with open arms.

You can volunteer at the expo for one day or the entire weekend. Volunteers at the expo will help direct participants to the right locations, guide participants to the right lines for packet pickup, hand out packets and race shirts, and even encourage friends and family members to make signs for their runner. These volunteers must be at least fifteen years old and will receive a piece of commemorative apparel and a snack per shift.

Volunteering opportunities are also available for the 5K and 10K events. You can help with getting participants into their corrals, hand out medals, and much more. Volunteers for these events must be at least twelve years old and will receive a commemorative piece of apparel and a snack per shift.

You can also volunteer at the main race itself. Choose from any of the races offered for the weekend in which you are interested. You may be asked to help fill water cups and hand them to the runners at the water stations. You may hand out gels to fuel the runners. You may even get to put the medal around the runners' necks at the finish line.

No matter what your job may be, know that all of the runners are very thankful for what you do, for you are truly making their race experience a great one. Volunteers must be at least twelve years of age (fifteen years of age at some locations) and will receive a commemorative piece of apparel, a snack per shift, and a one-day park ticket to the park of your choice.

If you are local, you have a great opportunity to volunteer at multiple events and work toward park tickets. For every hour spent volunteering, you receive a point. For every sixteen points earned, you get a one-day one-park ticket. Theme park tickets will be sent by mail within thirty days upon completion.

Each event also needs medical volunteers. These volunteers must be state-certified/licensed MDs, DOs, PAs, DPMs, ARNPs, RNs, ATCs, PTs, LMTs, PMs, or EMTs. Note that these volunteers may have very early or late shifts.

Do you have a large group interested in volunteering? There are great options for those with fifteen people or more. By registering as a group, you can ensure you all work at the same location and time. You will even receive advanced notice of upcoming events.

Once you have registered to volunteer, be sure to read any email or information that is sent to you. This will give you insight on what to bring, where to meet, and other important information. Do not forget your completed waiver and photo identification for when you arrive. Also, please don't forget sunscreen or a hat if it looks sunny or an umbrella and poncho if it looks rainy and, of course, comfortable shoes. Most important, bring your smile and words of encouragement for all the participants.

Volunteering opportunities are announced a few months prior to the event. Shifts are first come, first served, so register early. Visit **rundisney.com/volunteer/** for more information.

Deferring Registration

What happens if you get injured prior to your race? What if there is a family emergency? Or maybe if there is deployment? Unfortunately, your race registration is non-refundable and non-transferrable to another participant, but you might defer your registration to a later race. This must be done at least a month prior to the event and has a fee attached. Contact runDisney at **407-939-4786** to begin the process. Do note that there are limits as to how many runners can defer, so the sooner you can defer, the better.

If you choose to defer your race registration, it can only be deferred to the same race the following year. For example, if you sign up for the 2016 Princess Half-Marathon, you can only defer to a race during the 2017 Princess Half-Marathon weekend. A $35 fee does apply and is applied per transfer.

You can transfer your race registration to a different race during that same weekend. For example, you can transfer from the 2016 Walt Disney World 10K to the 2017 Walt Disney World Half-Marathon.

You are responsible for the difference between the two races and the transfer fee. If you transfer to a race that is less expensive, you may refunded the difference in fees.

To defer, you must fill out the form at runDisney.com, located on the registration tab for the race you are deferring. Once this is approved, you will receive a refund of your original race fee. Prior to registration for the next year's event, you will be given a unique link to register for the race weekend. Keep in mind that active.com fees will not be refunded, so you will ultimately be paying the fees twice.

If the race registration increases the next year, you will also pay the difference, up to $20. You will be informed of this fee by runDisney and given a time period to pay the additional fee.

Awards

Awards are available for each main event and the challenges. For the longer races, the top three male and female finishers will be given an award. Awards will also be given for the top three male and female wheelchair finishers.

It goes much farther. The third- to fifth-place male and female finishers for the military division will also receive awards. The overall male and female masters champions are awarded. Masters champions are those aged forty and older.

For everyone else, the top five male and female runners are given awards for the following age groups: 14-17, 18-24, 25-29, 30-34, 35-39, 40-44, 45-49, 50-54, 55-59, 60-64, 65-69, 70-74, 75-79, and 80+.

All awards for masters, military, and age groups will be mailed to you, so please allow some time for delivery.

Krista & Megan's Tips

- Register early! These races have been selling out faster and faster each year, some within one hour. You can sign up to receive a registration reminder when registration opens on the runDisney website, and we suggest that you put a reminder on your calendar.

- When looking for a race to update your proof of time, be sure to do a little research. Take a look at the course map, elevation, number of participants and even past reviews of the race.

- When you update your proof of time, it is highly recommended that you take a screen shot and print it in case any issues should arise later.

- In the past, Annual Passholders and Disney Vacation Club members have been allowed to register approximately one or two weeks early for some events providing peace of mind for the serious runner. There is a cap on how many can register early.

- The price of registration on the runDisney page does not include the Active.com fees, though you will be notified about these extra fees in the registration process. Be sure to factor in a little extra when budgeting for your races.

- Keep an eye on your name and birthdate (in particular) when registering for races. It is easy to switch the month and date of your birthdate in your hurry to register.

- Thinking about the *Runner's World* Challenge? It is a great option for runners wanting their experience to be one of a kind! Access to *Runner's World* editors and experts along with the greatest perk of all, the shortcut to the start line, makes it a great experience.

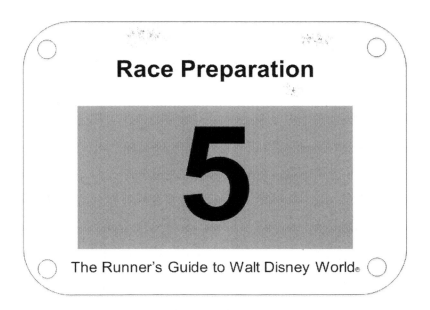

Race Preparation

5

The Runner's Guide to Walt Disney World®

You've signed up for your runDisney race. Now what?

It's time to train! Beyond getting in your mileage, there are many other aspects to training for a race of any distance. Here are some tips that will keep you motivated and ready to tackle your training.

Training

Did you know that runDisney has its very own training consultant? Former Olympian Jeff Galloway offers advice and training plans to all runDisney participants. Jeff created the run/walk/run method, which makes it possible for people of all ages, sizes, and fitness levels to train for and complete a runDisney event.

On the runDisney website, you can choose the training plan best for you. Whether it's your first long distance event or your fiftieth, Jeff has created a plan that will allow you to finish the race, and perhaps even finish in your fastest time yet. Plans vary from 18 to 28 weeks, depending on the length of your race, along with your running experience. The training plans are for the 10K distances and longer, but there are plans for other distances including the 5K on Jeff's website, **jeffgalloway.com**.

For those participating in the runDisney challenges such as Goofy's Race-and-a-Half Challenge, the Dopey Challenge, or the Glass Slipper Challenge, Jeff has created plans for you as well. These training plans are designed with the goal of finishing upright and making sure your body is prepared for back-to-back runs. A plus to Jeff's plans are that they can be downloaded to your calendar, compatible with Microsoft Outlook, Apple's iCal, and Google Calendar. By having your training plan on your calendar, there are no excuses on getting your training runs in.

Want to train with others? Be sure to check into local Galloway groups in your area. By using the run-walk-run method during training, you can train with others who run the same pace intervals. Your local Galloway group will help you measure or corroborate your pace, assign you to a training group with a group leader who will organize weekly runs, and provide you with a detailed training schedule to follow until race day. Yet one of the best advantages of a Galloway group is the social support you will receive. For more information, check out **jeffgalloway.com**.

For those interested, there are many other training plans available. Other great options include Hal Higdon and *Runner's World* Smart Coach. Be sure to do your research prior to choosing a training plan. Make sure the source is reputable and a plan you can handle.

If you are looking for more one-on-one coaching, check with your local running stores. They will have access to a list of qualified running coaches in your area. A common coaching certification is the Road Runners Club of America, **rrca.org**. Be sure to do a little research to ensure your coach is experienced and qualified.

Training For runDisney Events
(for beginners or time goal competitors)

Jeff Galloway
US Olympian
Official Training Consultant, runDisney
www.JeffGalloway.com

I designed each of the runDisney training schedules to prepare almost anyone for finishing the various events. The time-tested schedules have brought obese couch potatoes across the finish line and have helped seasoned veterans improve their personal best times.

Along with the schedules, you'll find a series of tools to keep you away from three things I despise: puking, pain and death.

The Magic Mile (MM) will tell you if your goal is realistic. Beginners need to monitor this to ensure they are fit enough to maintain a 16 min per mile pace to stay ahead of the "ballon ladies". Veterans can use the MM to choose a realistic goal and track progress. Be sure to use the MM guidelines to set up a safe, slow pace for long runs.

Long runs build endurance. One of the reasons for the high success rate of my programs is that you will actually cover the distance of the race event, 2-3 weeks beforehand. This bestows the physical and mental empowerment to go the distance on the big day. There is no long run pace that is too slow. Your only long run mission is to cover the distance.

My Run Walk Run method can be adjusted to avoid aches, pains and injury. The right strategy can allow each runner to do the training and finish the race—without exhaustion. This allows you to win your medal and then enjoy the parks afterward with friends and family. I have a supply of my Galloway timers at each event if you want one ($20).

Pacing guidelines use the MM to set a safe slow pace for long runs with suggested Run Walk Run strategies. Be sure to note the slowdown when hot: Run 30 sec slower per mile for every 5F temperature increase above 60F (20 sec/km slower for every 2.5C above 14C).

Many competitive runners have improved their times by following the time goal schedules at runDisney.com. Again, use the MM to set a realistic goal, and chart your progress. Be sure to attend my clinics on race weekend. I always have time for questions.

You Can Do It!

Nutrition

Another aspect of training is nutrition. It is important to fuel your body properly for your training runs and races. RunDisney has its very own nutritionist, Tara Gidus. Also known as the Diet Diva, Tara guides runners on how to stay healthy as they train. A runner herself, she gives real-world advice so that you can achieve maximum performance.

You can read Tara's blog posts regarding nutrition on the runDisney website, **RunDisney.com**. Tara covers topics such as how to fuel before a run, the importance of hydration, fueling for back-to-back races, and even some fantastic recipes. She also speaks at the Health and Fitness Expos, offering race weekend advice.

If you are training for a longer race such as a half-marathon or marathon, you will want to plan on fuel for partway through each race. RunDisney offers gels or chews at each half-marathon and marathon, though you should not forget your own fuel if these do not sit well with your stomach. Try out a few options during your training runs to determine what works best. Sport beans, gels, and chews are common, as are regular foods such as raisins, gummy candy, and bananas.

Support System

When embarking on your running journey, you should have a support system in place. This can include a friend or family member to hold you accountable to your training and to help with any future questions. If you like, besides your friends and family, there are some great running support groups online that can help you along the way.

Facebook.com not only keeps in touch with your family and friends, Facebook groups and pages are on the rise. These are great places to ask questions, get advice, and brag about your achievements. There are many groups for runDisney events, from individual races to running in general. When you log onto Facebook, you can search for terms such as the race name or runDisney. A list of groups will appear. Choose the ones you are interested in and join the group. (Some groups will require approval, but the administrators are usually very quick to accept your request.)

There are several Facebook groups where anyone can get support from other runners. Do keep in mind that there are no *official* runDisney Facebook groups. If you have a question that needs to be answered by runDisney specifically, please contact via email or phone.

Also, feel free to join us on our Facebook page at **facebook.com/RunnersGuideToWDW**

Looking for people in your town to run with? Then be sure to see if there are any running clubs. Go to your local gym or sporting goods/running stores and ask. They will be able to give you information to find runners who can encourage you with your training. Even better, you will make some great friends and maybe even run a runDisney race together.

Books, Blogs, and Podcasts

As you work toward your running goal, you may look for resources to help you on your journey. Various books, blogs, and podcasts are available to offer advice and information. Here are a few of our recommendations.

Books by Jeff Galloway

RunDisney's training consultant and run/walk/run method creator Jeff Galloway has a multitude of books full of fantastic information! His books include guides for all race distances (5K, 10K, half-marathon, and marathon) as well as a guide for his run/walk/run method. He also has a book devoted to the mental aspect of training, which includes advice for staying motivated as well as pushing through the tough miles. His wife Barbara has also co-authored a few books directed specifically toward women. These books are widely available at most local bookstores or from online retailers.

Books by Prominent Runners

At times a little motivation comes in reading the stories of others. Many prominent runners and Olympians have written books about their running journeys. Fan favorites include Bart Yasso, Christopher McDougall, Meb Keflezighi, Kristin Armstrong, and Dean Karnazes.

Another great resource is *Runner's World* magazine. Each month this magazine includes information for runners of all types. Information is also available on their website, as well as various book publications. *The Big Book of Training* is a great resource for all runners.

Podcasts

Downloading and listening to podcasts is a great way to get through those long runs. Below are a few favorites, but there truly is a podcast for everyone. From TV shows to fitness, advice to funny stories, do a little searching for one that will help make those miles fly by.

Jeff Galloway has his own edition of The Extra Mile podcast, which includes his training tips and even some of his running travels. Another favorite is the Let's Run Disney podcast. While there has been a hiatus in new episodes, the older episodes are still recommended. Keep your fingers crossed it will return.

The Mickey Miles podcast is another that has great information regarding runDisney races. They also host fun get together events (including dessert parties) during runDisney race weekends. The Marathon Show has a new host and is often at the runDisney events. Listen in to the show, then be on the lookout for Eddie at the upcoming race weekends.

Training Gear

When you begin your running journey, you may think that a good pair of shoes is all you need. While for some runners this may be true, many start to include additional running gear to enhance the running experience. Here is a look into options to consider.

Proper Running Shoes – This is the very first item you need to get when beginning your running journey. It is highly suggested that you go to your local running store to get properly fitted for running shoes. They will check your gait, foot type, arch, and running style to determine what shoe is best for you. They usually have a return policy if you find the shoe does not work for you. (If not, ask!) It is also recommended you get new shoes every 300-500 miles.

Sweat Wicking Clothing – Although you may have many cotton t-shirts and shorts lying around, they can be very uncomfortable as your mileage increases. Getting running clothes that wick away sweat will make your training runs much more comfortable. And ladies, be sure to get a proper sports bra that will help, not hinder, your run.

Garmin/GPS – As you begin to log your miles, you may want to start keeping track of your mileage each run. There are many options that will do this for you via GPS. Common items include a GPS watch (such as Garmin Forerunner, Nike+, or Timex) or a GPS app on your smartphone (such as MapMyRun, RunKeeper, or Nike+). With the watches, there are various price points, so be sure to do some research. Each watch offers different features, so you may want to ask other runners what they prefer.

Earphones – Whether outside or on the treadmill, sometimes music, audio books, or podcasts can get you through those training miles. Many find that the earphones that come with your phone are not the best for running. Thankfully, many companies have designed earphones that 'lock' into your ears and don't fall out when you sweat! Some are even wireless, keeping that pesky cord from bothering you on your run.

Visor/Hat/Headband – If you are training in the summer months or live in the south, many training runs include lots of sunshine. Wearing a hat or visor not only keeps the sun out of your face, but also helps curb sweat. A hat or visor is also great on rainy runs as it keeps the rain out of your face. Hats, visors, and headbands help control flyaway hair. As with everything, there are many options to choose from. Try to choose varieties that have sweat wicking capability.

Running Belt – As the mileage increases, you may want to bring more items along on your run. Running belts offer a place to store items such as your ID, keys, phone, fuel, etc. There are many types of running belts, ones that act more like a fanny pack and others that include hydration. Try on a few at your local running store to see what fit will be best for you as some sit on your hips and others are more around your waist.

Hydration System – It is so important for runners to stay hydrated, especially during the summer months. Bringing along water during your run ensures that you have hydration handy at all times. There are many ways to carry water with you including handheld water bottles, hydration belts (that carry a couple smaller water bottles), and hydration packs (that go on your back). It may take some trial and error to determine what option works best for you, but make sure you have water or electrolyte drinks with you on your runs.

Injury Prevention – A runner's worst nightmare is getting an injury that leaves them sidelined. At the onset of any aches or pains, be sure to treat them promptly. Common aches and pains can be treated with ice, and many runners choose to recover from a run with compression gear. If small aches continue to be a problem, items such as kiniseo tape and compression socks may help during a run. As always, consult your doctor if anything abnormal is occurring or if you have pain for multiple runs in a row.

Road ID/Safety Bracelet – Safety is extremely important during a training run or race. Along with being aware of your surroundings, run in areas that are well lit and safe. We also recommend wearing a bracelet (or similar item) that includes your medical information and person to contact. This way, if something does happen, medical professionals can act quickly. Road ID offers many options, including a phone app that will let your family member know where you are running.

Is it necessary to purchase or use all of this running gear? Absolutely not! What works for one runner may not work for another. Start by getting fitted for appropriate shoes at your local running store and go from there. Sweat wicking clothing is also important, but the rest of the gear is a matter of preference. We do highly suggest a safety bracelet and hydration system to ensure you are safe on your runs.

Krista & Megan's Tips

- When running your long runs, envision the race course. For example, if you are training for the Princess Half-Marathon, imagine that at Mile 5 you are entering Magic Kingdom or at Mile 11 you can see Epcot in view. This will help prepare you for your race.

- It is okay to miss some training runs! We all are busy, have things that come up, need a break, etc. However, if you find that you are missing many training runs (especially the longer runs), you may need to readjust your goals or distance.

- Training runs are the time to try out new things. Find out what fuel works, if you need to bring along a hydration belt, etc. Once you know what works, do the same on race day!

- There are many runDisney communities on Facebook and other social media platforms. Do your best to stay positive within the group and support one another, yet also be realistic. The running community as a whole is fantastic, so don't let items such as corral placement cause the community to break down!

- Planning on running in a costume? This popular option among many runDisney runners brings extra magic to the races! Be sure to get a training run or two in while wearing your costume, to make sure everything is good to go on race day.

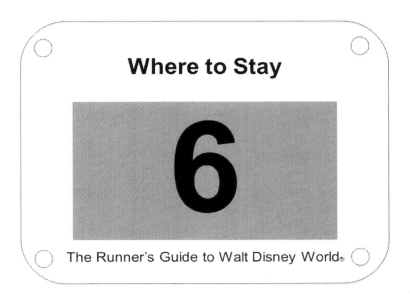

Where to Stay

6

The Runner's Guide to Walt Disney World®

Staying on Disney property is truly a magical experience. Not only are you well taken care of (in true Disney fashion), but there are also some great perks that come with staying on the property.

- Complimentary Disney transportation (bus, monorail, and ferry boat)
- Complimentary parking at Disney's theme parks (normally $17 per day)
- Easy access to parks, making midday breaks and naps possible, plus allowing parties to split up to go their independent ways
- Ability to make FastPass+ selections 60 days prior to arrival
- Charge privileges to your resort account for purchases throughout Disney
- Guaranteed entry to a Disney theme park (particularly important during busy holiday periods when filled-to-capacity parks often close to non-Disney resort guests)
- Extra Magic Hours whereby one of Disney's theme parks opens an hour early or up to three hours later than regular park hours exclusively for Disney resort guests

- Disney's Dining Plan that can save up to 30% per adult, if purchased, as part of your Magic Your Way Package
- Complimentary Titleist or Cobra club rentals with a full round of golf at any Disney golf course
- Package delivery from anywhere on-property directly to your resort
- Complimentary airport transportation via Disney's Magical Express buses
- The magic of Disney twenty-four hours a day

Disney offers four basic types of resorts: Value, Moderate, Deluxe and Deluxe Villas. Below is an approximate range of pricing per night.

Value Rooms - $100-200

Family Suites - $250-450

Moderate Rooms - $150-300

Deluxe Rooms - $300-1100

Deluxe Suites - $950-3200

Deluxe Villas - $300-2500

There are many types of rooms available within the Disney resorts. From standard rooms (ranging in square footage from 260 to 448) to suites (with up to 2,000 in square footage), there is a room for every type of family. There are also various room views available, which is the difference between looking out the window to a parking lot and looking out the window to Cinderella Castle.

Another room option is concierge level (also called club level). These rooms have access to a special keyed floor that includes a lounge that offers continental breakfast, afternoon snacks and beverages, evening appetizers, beer, wine, and after-dinner cordials and dessert. You also have access to concierge cast members (known as the Itinerary Planning Office) who will help you with dining reservations and much more.

> Based on the surveys from past runDisney participants:
>
> The top two Value Resorts are: Art of Animation and Pop Century
>
> The top two Moderate Resorts are: Port Orleans Riverside and Port Orleans French Quarter
>
> The top four Deluxe Resorts are: Contemporary Resort, Polynesian Resort, Wilderness Lodge, and Yacht Club

Runners interested in rooms that provide more space will enjoy the Deluxe Villa properties. These range from a deluxe studio (similar to a standard room) to grand three-bedroom villas. These villas also include kitchenettes or full-size kitchens for those wanting to bring their own food. A washer and dryer are available in one- and two-bedroom villas. While Disney Vacation Club members get priority, these villa properties open up approximately 7 months prior to arrival for the public.

The deluxe resorts also offer suites ranging from one-bedroom to presidential suites. These suites also have access to the concierge lounge and offer more room for those with large families. Keep in mind that these suites fill up quickly.

Since each resort on Disney property is unique, we have compiled information on each resort so that you can determine which resort is best for your family.

Host Resorts

All runDisney races are unique. Therefore, the host resorts for each race are also unique. Each race offers specific host resorts for the event. These resorts offer transportation to and from the expo, race, and other race events, which is by far the biggest. Also, in most instances of early morning races, the food court at the host resort will be open and serving pre-race food such as bagels and fruit.

You may be wondering how race transportation can be so important at a host resort. After all, you can just take a cab or drive your car to the race start. Yes, cabs can be taken to the start in the case of most morning races. However for the Wine & Dine Half-Marathon night race, runners are not allowed to take a cab directly to the race start. Runners must first board a bus at Epcot for Wine & Dine. If you are driving a car, you must park your car at this location and then board the bus. This extra step adds significant time to your pre-race plans. Runners at a host resort can board a bus directly to race starting lines from their resort, and after the post-race party, runners will find a bus that will transport them directly back to their resort. If you are considering a cab, please keep in mind that, due to traffic congestion, even a short cab ride can be very costly.

The only events that do not offer specific host resorts are Marathon Weekend and Princess Half-Marathon Weekend. Due to the large number of participants, all Disney resorts are host resorts and offer transportation to and from the expo and all race events. Also included during these race weekends is Shades of Green and Walt Disney World Swan and Dolphin.

Magic Kingdom Resorts

Imagine the convenience of being close to Cinderella Castle. For those with younger children (or the young at heart), these resorts in the Magic Kingdom area can't be beat. Magic Kingdom is just a monorail ride, ferry boat ride, or short walk away.

Disney's Contemporary Resort & Bay Lake Tower

This iconic resort was one of the first created at Walt Disney World. Its unique design stands out, especially as the monorail runs right through the center of the resort. With a contemporary feel (both inside the resort and the rooms themselves), this deluxe resort lives up to its name. The Contemporary Resort underwent extensive room refurbishment in 2013. Rooms have been freshly updated with a warm and welcoming contemporary décor. If you are looking for the best view of Cinderella Castle from your room, this resort offers just that.

Adjacent to the Contemporary Resort is Deluxe Villa property Bay Lake Tower, which offers accommodations from a small studio to a three-bedroom Grand Villa. These rooms are perfect for families looking for more space as well as runners who may wish to prepare their own food. All one-, two-, and three-bedroom villas have full kitchens.

The Contemporary Resort includes monorail service to Magic Kingdom and Epcot, a walking path to Magic Kingdom, and bus transportation to Hollywood Studios, Animal Kingdom, and Disney Springs. Ft. Wilderness and Wilderness Lodge resort are accessible via boat transportation.

Dining

Located in the Tower portion of the resort are three table service locations and one counter service location. (See Chapter 7 for more information.)

Amenities

As a deluxe resort, the Contemporary offers many amenities for you and your family to enjoy.

Included are two pools with a feature pool spanning over 6,500 square feet including a waterslide. There are also two whirlpool spas where you can relax after a long day in the parks. Kids can enjoy the playground area and arcade.

Your family can stay active with many recreational options. These include tennis, beach volleyball, water sports, fishing, boat rental, and more. There is also a health and fitness center for those wanting to get in a workout while on vacation. Guests looking for salon or spa services can take a quick monorail ride to the Grand Floridian.

For a real treat, enjoy the Electrical Water Pageant that runs every evening on the lake surrounding the Contemporary Resort. Head to the beach or even your balcony (depending upon your room type) for a great view! Check with your hotel concierge to verify the parade time each evening.

Race Course Proximity

A great benefit to the Contemporary resort is that participants in the Walt Disney World Marathon, Walt Disney World Half-Marathon, and Princess Half-Marathon will run by the Contemporary Resort. Watch the runners (from a distance) from your theme park view room, or head to the parking lot area to cheer them on as they run by.

You can also walk to Magic Kingdom to watch the runners on Main Street USA, allowing yourself a little time to sleep in. Then you can take the monorail to Epcot for the finish.

For the runners, staying at a monorail resort offers quick transportation to the race start. Hop on the monorail (making a switch at the Transportation and Ticket Center), then head to the staging area.

Room Types

This resort offers many room types, but the Theme Park View rooms truly can't be beat. Each room is 400 square feet in size and can accommodate up to five guests. All rooms have two queen-size beds or one king-size bed and a daybed. These rooms offer a large bathroom, though there is not a lot of storage space on the vanity. Included in the room is an alarm clock with mp3 player, coffee maker, hair dryer, in-room safe, iron and ironing board, telephone, flat-screen television, refrigerator, and wireless Internet.

Outside the main tower is a section of the resort known as the Garden Wing. These rooms are housed in a separate building. Although they may be cheaper in price, these rooms require more walking to get to the monorail, bus transportation, and dining locations. However, they can provide a great value for guests who want to be near Magic Kingdom and on the monorail.

In the main tower, there are two basic room types: Bay Lake View and Theme Park View. The Bay Lake View rooms are on the backside of the tower, giving views of Bay Lake and the pool. The Theme Park Views are a must-do. Imagine standing on your balcony in the evening, watching the Wishes fireworks show in Magic Kingdom from the comfort of your own room. These rooms are the closest to Magic Kingdom throughout the Walt Disney World Resort.

The Contemporary Resort also offers concierge level rooms as well as many types of suites. The one-bedroom suites are 1,428 square feet and include a bedroom, bathroom, and living room area. A standard room can be added to this suite to make it a two-bedroom suite. Also available is the Vice-Presidential Suite at 1,985 square feet. Included is a living area, two bedrooms and three bathrooms. The grandest suite is the Presidential Suite, which is 2,061 square feet and includes a kitchen and wet bar, a living room, two bedrooms, and three bathrooms.

Bay Lake Tower at Disney's Contemporary Resort

At Bay Lake Tower, there are deluxe studios, one- and two-bedroom villas, and a few Grand Villas. The Deluxe Studios are 356 square feet and are similar to the rooms at the Contemporary. However, these rooms also include a kitchenette with a toaster and microwave. These rooms accommodate up to four guests.

The one-bedroom villas are 727 square feet and include a separate master bedroom and bathroom. These rooms feature a full-sized kitchen that includes a larger refrigerator, sink, oven, stove, and microwave as well as plates, flatware, glasses, pots, pans, and more. The master bedroom includes a king-size bed, and the living area includes a queen-size sleeper sofa. This room accommodates up to five guests.

The two-bedroom villas are 1,080 square feet and combine the deluxe studio with the one-bedroom villa. These rooms can accommodate up to eight guests.

There are also a few three-bedroom or Grand Villas that accommodate up to twelve guests. These villas span multiple levels and offer breathtaking views of Magic Kingdom and the Seven Seas Lagoon.

Disney's Polynesian Village Resort

Travel to the Seven Seas and enjoy the island décor at the Polynesian Resort. With dark wood tones and lush gardens, you truly feel that you have traveled to the islands in this deluxe resort. Enter the lobby, where you will be greeted with an "Aloha." Take a walk on the white sand beach, lie in the hammock, or sway in the island breeze while enjoying a view of Cinderella's Castle from across the bay.

The Polynesian Resort includes monorail service to Magic Kingdom and Epcot, ferry boat transportation to Magic Kingdom, and bus transportation to Hollywood Studios, Animal Kingdom, and Disney Springs.

Throughout 2015, the Polynesian Resort is underwent a major renovation. The rooms were given a much-needed, bright, new look. Various areas of the grounds were revamped, bungalow villas were added over the Seven Seas Lagoon. Areas around the resort, including the smaller pool area, will continue to be worked on through early 2016.

Dining

Located in the Great Ceremonial House, the Polynesian resort offers a quick-service restaurant, along with two table-service locations. There is also a special dinner show in the form of a luau located at this resort. (See Chapter 7 for more information.)

This resort also has a bar, lounge, and 24-hour in-room dining.

Amenities

The Polynesian Resort offers an array of great amenities for runners and families alike.

The Lava Pool has historically been one of the best pools on Disney property and underwent an elaborate refurbishment which further enhanced its features. With a forty-foot-high volcano, waterfall, waterslide, and play area for the little ones, everyone in the family will find something to keep them smiling at this pool. There is another smaller pool on the property (Polynesian East Pool), which is commonly referred to as the quiet pool. This pool will continue to be worked on through early 2016.

There are many great recreational opportunities available at this resort including bike rentals, fishing, jogging trails, an arcade, and more. You can also take specialty cruises on the Seven Seas Lagoon, with the Wishes Fireworks Cruise being one of the most popular. The marina also offers boat rentals, from Sea Raycers to canoes.

Those staying at the Polynesian Resort can use the same fitness center and hot tub as the Grand Floridian. This fitness center is open 24/7 and is about a fifteen-minute walk from the resort.

You can also head to the Senses Spa at the Grand Floridian for a truly relaxing experience. Enjoy a massage, facial, manicure, pedicure, and more: a great treat after your race.

Lilo's Playhouse is for those aged three to twelve to enjoy. Let the kids play with their friends and cast members while you enjoy a night out. This is open from 4:30 p.m. to midnight for a charge of $15 per child per hour, with a two-hour minimum. Guests do not have to be staying at the Polynesian to use Club Disney.

Race Course Proximity

A great benefit is that participants in the Walt Disney World Marathon, Walt Disney World Half-Marathon, and Princess Half-Marathon will run near the Polynesian Resort. If you walk through the parking lot to the service road, you can cheer on the runners as they go by.

Spectators can also take the monorail to Magic Kingdom to watch the runners on Main Street USA then take the monorail to Epcot for the finish. This allows the family a little extra time to sleep in.

For the runners, staying at a monorail resort offers quick transportation to the race start, specifically for the races that begin at Epcot. Hop on the monorail (making a switch at the Transportation and Ticket Center) then head to the staging area. Those staying at the Polynesian can choose to walk to the Transportation and Ticket Center and get on the monorail to Epcot from there.

Room Types

All rooms at the Polynesian underwent extensive renovation in 2014. The Polynesian Resort offers a few room types, but the Theme Park View rooms are the best in the resort. It overlooks a white sand beach, and across the Seven Seas Lagoon you can see Cinderella Castle and Space Mountain. However, these views now also include the bungalows.

Each room in the Polynesian Resort is 404 square feet and can accommodate up to five guests. All rooms have two queen-size beds and a daybed. These rooms offer a large bathroom. Included in the room is an alarm clock with mp3 player, coffee maker, hair dryer, in-room safe, iron and ironing board, telephone, flat-screen television, refrigerator, and wireless Internet.

There are three basic room views: Standard View, Lagoon View, and Theme Park View. A few of the Standard View rooms may offer views of the parking lot and may be near the monorail line, which may be noisy. Also, the Theme Park View rooms offer a view across the Seven Seas Lagoon, which means that Space Mountain may be more prominent than Cinderella Castle. However, the view of the Wishes fireworks show from the beach is quite amazing.

One main thing to consider at the Polynesian Resort is having a balcony. The first floor rooms only offer a patio that opens directly to the grounds. The third floor rooms offer a balcony, whereas the second floor rooms have no balcony. (Keep in mind, a room request is just that: a request and not a guarantee.)

The Polynesian Resort also offers concierge level rooms and many types of suites. First is the Honeymoon Room, which is slightly larger than a standard room and includes a whirlpool tub. The Princess Suite includes two bedrooms, two bathrooms, and a living area. (There is also a one-bedroom Princess option.) The Ambassador Suites are 1,513 square feet and include two bedrooms and three bathrooms along with a living area. The ultimate suite is the King Kamehameha, a two-story suite spanning 1,863 square feet. It includes two bedrooms, two-and-a-half bathrooms, living area, parlor, and kitchen.

Disney's Polynesian Villas & Bungalows

This Disney Vacation Club property opened in April 2015 and provides additional offerings for guests looking for more space in the Magic Kingdom area. This property offers deluxe studios and bungalows.

Deluxe studios will sleep up to five with one queen-size bed, one queen sleeper sofa, and one twin pull-down bed.

The bungalows are a unique addition to the Polynesian Resort. With room for up to 8 guests, this 2-bedroom, 2-bathroom bungalow sits atop the Seven Seas Lagoon. Each includes a private back deck and plunge pool. The bungalows also include living, kitchen and dining areas, a washer and dryer and views of the lagoon and Cinderella Castle.

Disney's Grand Floridian Resort & Spa and Villas

Transport yourself to the turn of the century with Victorian-inspired themes throughout this flagship deluxe resort. The white buildings and red roofs are familiar sights to many. Enter the lobby to view a giant crystal chandelier and listen to the music of the piano or jazz band.

The Grand Floridian Resort & Spa includes monorail service to Magic Kingdom and Epcot, ferry boat service to Magic Kingdom, and bus transportation to Hollywood Studios, Animal Kingdom, and Disney Springs.

Dining

The Grand Floridian Resort and Spa offers many famous restaurants. From five-diamond restaurants to character meals, you and your family will find any type of cuisine you desire. (See Chapter 7 for more information.)

This resort also has a bar, lounge, and 24-hour in-room dining.

Amenities

There are many great amenities for adults and children alike. Numerous options abound, whether you would like to rent a watercraft, take a dip in the pool, play in the arcade, or rent a poolside cabana. Each evening, a movie under the stars is available for your enjoyment.

The Pirate Adventure Cruise is a unique opportunity for those aged four to twelve, where they can put on a pirate bandana and search for buried treasure. While on your pirate ship, you will make "ports of call" (other resort marinas) while searching for your treasure and listening to The Legend of Gasparilla.

For a truly relaxing experience, enjoy the Senses Spa. If you are in need of some pampering, look no further than this world-class spa. There are many body treatments, skin care, massages, and more that will make you feel rejuvenated. There is also a fitness center for those wanting to get in a workout or two.

Race Course Proximity

A great benefit is that participants in the Walt Disney World Marathon, Walt Disney World Half-Marathon and Princess Half-Marathon will run near the Grand Floridian Resort. If you walk through the parking lot to the back service road, you can cheer on the racers as they run by.

You can also take the monorail to Magic Kingdom to watch the runners on Main Street USA, and then take the monorail to Epcot for the finish.

For the runners, staying on a monorail resort offers quick transportation to the race start, specifically the races that begin at Epcot. Hop on the monorail (making a switch at the Transportation and Ticket Center) then head to the staging area.

Room Types

There are many room types available at the Grand Floridian Resort. All rooms offer views of the pool, Seven Seas Lagoon, or theme park. There are rooms in the main building (all concierge level) and in the outer buildings. Throughout 2014, the rooms received a much needed renovation.

Rooms are at least 448 square feet and can accommodate up to five people. All rooms have two queen-size beds or king bed, and some rooms offer a daybed. These rooms offer a large bathroom. Included in the room is an alarm clock with mp3 player, coffee maker, hair dryer, in-room safe, iron and ironing board, telephone, flat-screen television, refrigerator, robes, and wireless Internet.

Deluxe rooms in the outer buildings offer a little more room for those larger families. There are also larger rooms available in the main building. The Grand Floridian offers many types of suites as well both in the main building and outer buildings. There are also concierge level rooms available in the main and outer buildings.

The Grand Floridian Resort offers twenty-five suites. In the Outer Building, there are one- and two-bedroom suites. The two-bedroom suites are essentially two standard rooms joined by a living room. The main building offers various suites. The Victorian Suite is 1,083 square feet and includes a bedroom, bathroom, and living area. There are two suites with 1,690 square feet: the Walt Disney Suite and Roy O. Disney Suite. Both offer two bedrooms, two-and-a-half bathrooms, and a living area. The difference between the two suites is the décor. Looking for another option? Choose the Grand Suite at 2,220 square feet, which includes two bedrooms, two bathrooms, living area, kitchen, and five balconies. In this spacious suite, there is plenty of room for large families!

The Villas at Disney's Grand Floridian Resort and Spa

This Disney Vacation Club property opened October 2013 and provides additional offerings for guests looking for more space in the Magic Kingdom area. This property offers studios and one- and two-bedroom villas with luxurious furnishings. In all room types, guests can choose from a standard or lake view.

Deluxe studios will sleep up to five with one queen-size bed, one queen sleeper sofa, and one twin pull-down bed.

One-bedroom villas also sleep up to five but offer additional space and privacy. Accommodations include one king-size bed, one queen sleeper sofa, and one twin pull-down bed. One-bedroom villas include a full kitchen with living room and a separate bedroom. A stackable washer and dryer are located in each unit.

Two-bedroom villas are perfect for large or multi-generational families and sleep up to nine. These two-bedroom villas include two full-sized bathrooms, one king bed, one queen bed, one queen sleeper sofas, and two twin pull-down beds. These units also include a full kitchen, living area, and a stackable washer and dryer.

Disney's Wilderness Lodge and Villas

Travel back to a 1900s national park in this deluxe resort in the woods. From its wooden exterior, totem pole-lined lobby, and working geyser, the Wilderness Lodge stays true to its theme. This property also includes Deluxe Villas within the same resort.

The Wilderness Lodge offers ferry boat service to Magic Kingdom, Ft. Wilderness, and Contemporary Resort, as well as bus transportation to Epcot, Hollywood Studios, Animal Kingdom, and Disney Springs.

This resort offers the convenience of being close to Magic Kingdom with a smaller price tag. Do keep in mind that the only transportation to the park is by ferry boat.

Wilderness Lodge will be undergoing an extensive refurbishment beginning October 2015 through 2017. This includes enhancements to the Hidden Springs pool, closed pathways and various additions to the resort. Keep this in mind when planning your race plans for 2016.

Dining

From a hootin' and hollerin' time to a serene experience, there are many food options at the Wilderness Lodge. (See Chapter 7 for more information.)

This resort also has a bar, lounge, and 24-hour in-room dining.

Amenities

The Wilderness Lodge offers many great amenities including an arcade, small beach, recreation, and as a newly refurbished pool and play area. Perhaps your family would like to rent a boat and do some fishing or rent a bicycle and go for a spin. You can even get a "ranger"-led tour of the property. There is also a fitness center for those wishing to get in a workout during their stay.

The theming of this resort continues outside. Follow the bubbling spring in the lobby as it becomes a waterfall into the feature pool. Silver Creek Springs, the main pool, includes a waterslide and hot tub and is nestled in the surrounding trees. There is also a quiet pool (Hidden Springs) with another hot tub perfect for a post-race soak.

The Cub's Den is available from 4:30 p.m. to midnight for potty-trained children aged three to twelve. This way the adults can have a night to themselves while the children play video games, experience arts and crafts, and watch their favorite Disney movies.

A couple can't-miss items include the nightly Electrical Water Pageant. Watch King Neptune and his court make their way across the water in a musical revue. Another must-see is the Fire Rock Geyser, which erupts every hour.

Room Types

With this resort, there are many room types: standard rooms, suites, and villas. Room views include standard, woods, and courtyard. A few rooms do have glimpses of Magic Kingdom, although this is rare. To see the Magic Kingdom fireworks from Wilderness Lodge, book a Woods View room and request a high floor overlooking Otter Pond.

Standard rooms have 356 square feet of space and can accommodate up to four people. All rooms have two queen-size beds or one queen bed with a set of bunk beds. These rooms offer wireless Internet, a large bathroom, an alarm clock with mp3 player, coffee maker, hair dryer, in-room safe, iron and ironing board, telephone, flat-screen television, and refrigerator.

The Wilderness Lodge also offers club level rooms and many types of suites. The Vice-Presidential Suite is 885 square feet and includes one bedroom, one-and-a-half baths, living room, and dining area. The Presidential Suite is 1,000 square feet and includes one bedroom, one-and-a-half baths, and living area.

The Villas at Disney's Wilderness Lodge

Deluxe Villas provide a variety of options, including deluxe studios and one- and two-bedroom villas. The deluxe studios are 356 square feet and are similar to the rooms at Wilderness Lodge. However, these rooms also feature a kitchenette with a toaster and microwave. These rooms accommodate up to four guests.

The one-bedroom villas are 727 square feet and include a separate master bedroom and bathroom. A full-sized kitchen includes a larger refrigerator, sink, oven, stove, and microwave as well as plates, flatware, glasses, pots, pans, and more. The master bedroom includes a king-size bed, and the living area includes a queen-size sleeper sofa. This room accommodates up to four guests.

The two-bedroom villas are 1,080 square feet and combine the deluxe studio with the one-bedroom villa. These rooms can accommodate up to eight guests.

All one- and two-bedroom deluxe villas include a washer and dryer.

Disney's Fort Wilderness Resort and Campground

Looking for a truly rustic experience? Then Fort Wilderness Resort may be just the thing for your family. Bring your own tent, travel trailer, or RV, or stay in a cabin on property.

Fort Wilderness Resort offers ferry boat service to Magic Kingdom and bus transportation to Epcot, Hollywood Studios, Animal Kingdom, and Disney Springs.

Dining

Fort Wilderness Resort offers a great table-service restaurant and two fun dinner shows that the entire family will enjoy. (See Chapter 7 for more information.)

Amenities

Fort Wilderness Resort offers many special amenities as most guests bring their own accommodations. Throughout the area are comfort stations offering air conditioning, private restrooms, showers, ice machines, and laundry facilities. There is even a trading post that carries groceries, propane tanks, and more.

For those wanting to watch a movie, there is a video rental location. Your family can also rent an electric cart that can fit up to four adults.

Since this is a campground, pets are allowed for resort guests staying in RVs. Pets (other than service animals) are not allowed in the cabins. If you wish to have your pet watched while you explore the parks, Best Friends Pet Care is available and includes accommodations, activities and more for your pet.
BestFriendsPetCare.com

In terms of recreation, the possibilities are endless. Tennis, volleyball, fishing, playground, video games, bike, and watercraft rentals: there is so much for your family to enjoy. There is even a pool, called the Swimmin' Hole, as well as a waterslide and hot tub.

Head to the Tri-Circle-D Ranch to see the horses. It's the only ranch on Walt Disney World property. You can ride horses and ponies and even get a carriage or sleigh ride. Join Chip 'n' Dale at night for a campfire, singing, s'mores, and a movie under the stars.

Room Types

There are many campsite types for your tent, trailer, or RV. Every campsite includes water, electricity, a charcoal grill, picnic table, high speed Internet access, and cable television connection.

A basic tent or pop-up camper campsite includes the above. It can accommodate one pop-up camper plus a tent, or two tents.

A full-hook up campsite can accommodate one RV plus a tent or two tents. Equipment must not be larger than 10' x 60'.

A preferred campsite is in a premium location and includes an upgraded charcoal grill and picnic table. It accommodates one RV plus a tent, or two tents. This campsite can accommodate the largest motorhomes and trailers, and pets are allowed in some areas.

A premium campsite includes the same as a preferred campsite, along with an extra-large concrete parking pad for your trailer or RV. It can accommodate one RV plus a tent, or two tents.

For those wanting accommodations in this area but not in a trailer, RV, or tent, there are cabins available. These cabins accommodate up to six people and include a double bed, one set of bunk beds, and a pull-down double bed in the living area. There is also one full bathroom, a dining table, and a fully equipped kitchen with a refrigerator, stove, microwave, dishwasher, coffeemaker, toaster, dishes, and pots and pans. These cabins are air-conditioned and include cable television, high speed Internet, a charcoal grill, picnic table, and daily housekeeping.

> Find a resort that meets your needs and those of the other travelers with you. The people with me do make a difference - kids/no kids, runners/spectators, and help shape which resort we pick.
>
> *Andrea, VA*

Epcot Resorts

For those who love wandering the countries in Epcot, the Yacht Club, Beach Club, and Boardwalk Inn are just for you! With easy walking access to Epcot (through the International Gateway), the location can't be beat. There are also walking paths and ferry boats to Hollywood Studios, as well as access to the Swan and Dolphin hotels. For races that finish at Epcot, this location is ideal. Runners will need a park ticket to walk through the park and back to their resorts. Keep in mind, if you do not have a park hopper ticket, then you will need to spend your race day at Epcot.

Disney's Beach Club Resort and Villas

In this New England-style resort, enjoy a close proximity to Epcot while overlooking Crescent Lake and the Boardwalk. This deluxe resort boasts the best pool on Disney property (Stormalong Bay), a sort of mini-waterpark.

The Beach Club offers a walking path to Epcot, ferry boat service to Hollywood Studios, and bus transportation to Magic Kingdom, Animal Kingdom, and Disney Springs. The walking path from Epcot is what makes this resort a fantastic option after a race that finishes at Epcot. Just make sure you have your park ticket to walk through the park.

Dining

The Beach Club offers a counter service, fun table service, and a character meal. Due to the close proximity to the Yacht Club and Boardwalk, there are many other offerings to experience. (See Chapter 7 for more information.)

Amenities

The Beach Club offers many great amenities for families and runners. The most spectacular is the mini-water park pool, Stormalong Bay. Enjoy three acres of water fun, including a shipwreck slide, sand bottom pool, lazy river, and a zero-entry or walk-in kiddie pool.

The Ship Shape Health Club is great for those wanting to get in a workout or relax with a massage. There is also a sauna and steam room as well as body and hair treatments. Open 24/7, this health club is a great option for runners who want to get in a pre- or post-race workout.

For the adults wanting a night out, the Sandcastle Club offers an activity center for potty-trained kids aged three to twelve. Open from 4:30 p.m. to midnight, the center has video games, arts and crafts, movies, and more. Dinner is included. Guests can make reservations by visiting their hotel concierge or calling 407-WDW-DINE.

Many forms of recreation are available. Rent a bike for a trip around the Boardwalk. Take a fishing excursion on Crescent Lake. Rack up points at the arcade. Enjoy a game or two of tennis or volleyball. Take a specialty cruise and watch Illuminations. There is something for everyone.

Race Course Proximity

A great benefit is that participants in the Walt Disney World 10K, Walt Disney World Marathon, Princess 10K and Wine & Dine Half-Marathon will run near the Beach Club Resort. Watch the runners (from a distance) from your water view room, or head to the Boardwalk area to cheer them as they run by.

If a race is finishing in Epcot, you may walk through Epcot (entering through the International Gateway) to get to the finish line in the parking lot area, but you must have a valid theme park ticket to enter the park.

Room Types

The Beach Club offers various room types and room views including garden and pool views. However, the pool and water views can't be beat, especially for a great view of the Marathon and Wine & Dine routes. The Beach Club also offers deluxe villas for those looking for more space.

Standard rooms are 400 square feet, and some rooms can accommodate up to five people. All rooms have two queen-size beds or a king bed, and some rooms feature a daybed. These rooms offer a large bathroom. Included in the room is an alarm clock with mp3 player, coffee maker, hair dryer, in-room safe, iron and ironing board, telephone, flat-screen television, refrigerator, robes, and wireless Internet.

The Beach Club also offers club level rooms and many types of suites. (Note: There are a few deluxe rooms that offer 133 more square feet than a standard room. These are also concierge level.) The one-bedroom suites are 726 square feet and include a bedroom, bathroom, and small parlor. The two-bedroom suites include two bedrooms, two bathrooms, and a living area. The Vice-Presidential Nantucket Suite is 996 square feet and includes one bedroom, one-and-a-half baths, and living area. The grandest suite is the Presidential Newport Suite at 2,200 square feet. With two bedrooms, two-and-a-half bathrooms, living area, small kitchen, and sitting areas, there is room for everyone.

Disney's Beach Club Villas

Deluxe Villas at Disney's Beach Club offer deluxe studios and one- and two-bedroom villas. The deluxe studios are 356 square feet and are similar to the rooms at Wilderness Lodge, except that these rooms also include a kitchenette with a toaster and microwave. These rooms accommodate up to four guests.

The one-bedroom villas are 726 square feet and include a separate master bedroom and bathroom. Also included is a full-sized kitchen with a larger refrigerator, sink, oven, stove, and microwave, and plates, flatware, glasses, pots, pans, and more. The master bedroom includes a king-size bed, and the living area includes a queen-size sleeper sofa. This room accommodates up to four guests.

The two-bedroom villas comprise 1,083 square feet and combine the deluxe studio with the one-bedroom villa. These rooms can accommodate up to eight guests.

Disney's Yacht Club Resort

Adjoining the Beach Club, the Yacht Club shares many of the same amenities, but in a slightly more secluded venue.

The Yacht Club offers a walking path to Epcot, ferry boat service to Hollywood Studios, and bus transportation to Magic Kingdom, Animal Kingdom, and Disney Springs. The walking path from Epcot is what makes this resort a fantastic option after a race that finishes at Epcot. Just make sure you have your park ticket so you can walk through the park.

Dining

With its close proximity to the Beach Club and Boardwalk, there are many opportunities for great dining with your family. (See Chapter 7 for more information.)

Amenities

Since this resort adjoins the Beach Club, all amenities are shared. (See earlier Beach Club section for a listing.) The same is true for race course proximity.

Room Types

The Yacht Club offers various room types and room views including garden and pool views. However, the pool and water views can't be beat, especially for a great view of the Marathon and Wine & Dine race routes.

Standard rooms are 400 square feet, and some rooms can accommodate up to five people. All rooms have two queen-size beds or a king bed, and some rooms feature a daybed. These rooms offer a large bathroom. Included in the room is an alarm clock with mp3 player, coffee maker, hair dryer, in-room safe, iron and ironing board, telephone, flat-screen television, refrigerator, robes, and wireless Internet.

The Yacht Club also offers club level rooms as well as many types of suites. (Note: There are a few deluxe rooms that offer 254 more square feet than a standard room. These are also concierge level.) The Turret two-bedroom suite is 1,160 square feet and includes two bedrooms, two bathrooms, living area, and dining area. The Presidential and Admiral Suites are 2,017 square feet and offer two bedrooms, two-and-a-half bathrooms, and two living areas, dining room, and small kitchen. The largest suite is the Captain's Suite at 2,374 square feet for a large foyer, two bedrooms, two-and-a-half bathrooms, living area, sitting area, and dining room.

Disney's Boardwalk Inn and Villas

Head back to a 1930s seacoast in this recreation of an Atlantic boardwalk. Walk along the Boardwalk to experience the great entertainment and music or look out your balcony for views of Epcot.

The Boardwalk Inn offers a walking path to Epcot, ferry boat service to Hollywood Studios, and bus transportation to Magic Kingdom,

Animal Kingdom, and Disney Springs. Like the Beach Club and Yacht Club, the walking path from Epcot is what makes this resort a fantastic option after a race that finishes at Epcot. Just make sure you have your park ticket to walk through the park.

Dining

The Boardwalk is a great place to experience many cuisines. This resort is close to the Beach Club and Yacht Club, so you can take advantage of those restaurants as well. (See Chapter 7 for more information.)

Amenities

This deluxe resort offers many amenities to its guests. The Muscle and Bustle Health Club includes a fitness center, massage therapy, and a sauna.

There are three pools available for your family to enjoy. The Luna Park pool is the largest and includes a waterslide. There are also two quiet pools to enjoy.

Your family can rent bikes to ride up and down the Boardwalk. The Community Hall is a great place to play a board game or two, and there are even some arts and crafts. Take a fishing trip along Crescent Lake, or climb the playground located near Luna Park pool. Your family can also rent boats to ride along Crescent Lake or take a specialty Illuminations cruise. Play a round of tennis or eighteen holes of miniature golf at Fantasia Gardens.

The Boardwalk Area also has one of the best jogging trails on Disney property, so don't miss out.

Race Course Proximity

A great benefit is that participants in the Walt Disney World 10K, Walt Disney World Marathon, Princess 10K and Wine & Dine Half-Marathon will run near the Boardwalk Inn. Watch the runners from your water view room or head to the Boardwalk area to cheer them as they run by.

If a race is finishing in Epcot, you may walk through Epcot (entering through the International Gateway) to get to the finish line in the parking lot area, but you must have a valid theme park ticket to enter the park.

Room Types

The Boardwalk offers two room views, standard and water view. The water views are excellent, overlooking the Boardwalk, Crescent Lake, and Epcot. These views are also great for watching runners along the Marathon and Wine & Dine route. The Boardwalk Inn also offers deluxe villas.

Standard rooms are 434 square feet, and some rooms accommodate up to five people. All rooms have two queen-size beds or a king bed with a daybed. These rooms offer a large bathroom, an alarm clock with mp3 player, coffee maker, hair dryer, in-room safe, iron and ironing board, telephone, flat-screen television, refrigerator, and wireless Internet.

The Boardwalk Inn also offers concierge level rooms and many types of suites. The two-storied Garden Suites are 915 square feet and include a loft, two bathrooms, and a living area that converts to another sleeping area. There are two-bedroom suites of 1,288 square feet that include two-and-a-half bathrooms, a living area, and a parlor. The Vice Presidential Sonora Suite includes two bedrooms, two-and-a-half bathrooms, and a large living area. The largest suite is the Presidential Steeplechase Suite at 2,170 square feet for two bedrooms, two-and-a-half bathrooms, a living area, dining area, and service kitchen.

Disney's Boardwalk Villas

Boardwalk Villas provide a variety of options such deluxe studios and one- and two-bedroom villas. The deluxe studios are 412 square feet and are similar to the rooms at Wilderness Lodge. However, these rooms include a kitchenette with a toaster and microwave. These rooms accommodate up to four guests.

The one-bedroom villas are 814 square feet and include a separate master bedroom and bathroom. Also included is a full-size kitchen with a larger refrigerator, sink, oven, stove, and microwave as well as plates, flatware, glasses, pots, pans, and more. The master bedroom includes a king-size bed, and the living area includes a queen-size sleeper sofa. This room accommodates up to four guests.

The two-bedroom villas are 1,236 square feet and combine the deluxe studio with the one-bedroom villa. These rooms can accommodate up to eight guests.

There are also a few three-bedroom or Grand Villas that accommodate up to twelve guests. A few of these villas span over two levels.

Disney's Caribbean Beach Resort

Sail away to a tropical paradise at Caribbean Beach Resort. Enjoy white sand beaches, brightly colored buildings, and palm trees swaying in the breeze at this moderate resort.

Caribbean Beach offers bus transportation to all the parks: Magic Kingdom, Epcot, Hollywood Studios, Animal Kingdom, and Disney Springs.

Dining

This moderate resort offers a counter-service food court and table-service restaurant. (See Chapter 7 for more information.)

Amenities

Caribbean Beach offers several amenities for your family to enjoy. The main pool (located near Old Port Royale) includes two waterslides, water cannons, and hot tubs. And don't miss out on the six heated pools throughout the resort. Laundry services are available. Bikes and watercraft can be rented for some fun recreation. There are also beach volleyball courts and a great jogging trail throughout the resort for those looking to be even more active on vacation. You can also try your hand at your favorite arcade games.

Room Types

Caribbean Beach offers some great room types just for families. From water views to pirate rooms, there is something for everyone. The preferred rooms are closer to the food court and bus stops. For those with young children, a preferred room is a must, as this resort is very spread out.

Standard rooms are 300 square feet and can accommodate up to four people. All rooms have two double beds or a king bed. These rooms offer a bathroom with separate vanity area. Included in the room is a coffee maker, hair dryer, in-room safe, iron and ironing board, telephone, flat-screen television, refrigerator, and wireless Internet.

For those families wanting a swashbuckling experience, be sure to choose a pirate-themed room. The beds are shaped like pirate ships among other pirate décor.

Disney's Art of Animation Resort

Walt Disney World's newest resort brings your favorite animated movies to life. This Value Plus resort boasts great design as the

Lion King, Finding Nemo, Cars, and the Little Mermaid welcome you home.

Art of Animation offers bus transportation to all parks: Magic Kingdom, Epcot, Hollywood Studios, Animal Kingdom, and Disney Springs.

Dining

Although there is only one dining location on property, it is sure to keep your family satisfied. Quite possibly the best food court at Walt Disney World, so everyone will find something they love. (See Chapter 7 for more information.)

Amenities

Art of Animation amenities are abundant. Enjoy three pools, from the feature Big Blue Pool near the Finding Nemo area to the smaller Cozy Cone Pool in the Cars area and The Little Mermaid Pool. There is also a fun schoolyard wet play area for kids to enjoy. Watch a movie under the stars in the Lion King area of Art of Animation. An arcade is located in the main building and Ping Pong tables are located pool side. A cozy playground is located in the Lion King area.

Room Types

Art of Animation is unique as only two room types are available. However, there are multiple themes available.

Standard rooms are 277 square feet and can accommodate up to four people. These rooms have two double beds as well as a hair dryer, in-room safe, iron and ironing board, telephone, flat-screen television, refrigerator, and wireless Internet. All standard rooms at Art of Animation have a Little Mermaid theme.

Family suites are 565 square feet and can accommodate up to six people. These rooms have three separate sleeping areas, including a master bedroom with queen-size bed, a full-size sleeper sofa with memory foam mattress, and a full-size convertible table bed with memory foam mattress, two full-size bathrooms, a kitchenette that includes a mini-fridge, microwave and coffeemaker, a table and chairs, two flat panel TVs, in-room wall safe, voice mail, and wireless Internet access. These family suites have Lion King, Finding Nemo, or Cars themes.

Want to stay at Art of Animation when it's not a host resort? As long as either Pop Century or Art of Animation is a host resort, you are in the clear. Head toward the back of the property and cross the bridge that connects the two resorts. Once you are at the other property, you can board transportation to any of the race events.

Disney's Pop Century Resort

With a bright salute to twentieth-century icons, this value resort brings your favorite music, fads, toys, and more to life.

Pop Century offers bus transportation to all the parks: Magic Kingdom, Epcot, Hollywood Studios, Animal Kingdom, and Disney Springs.

Dining

This resort only offers a counter-service food court. There are many choices, sure to delight even the pickiest eater. (See Chapter 7 for more information.)

Amenities

Pop Century offers three pools, the featured Hippy Dippy pool (shaped like a flower) in the '60s section and the smaller Bowling and Computer pools in the '50s and '90s sections, respectively. For those wanting to try their hand at video games, the arcade is a great place to hang out. There is also a playground for kids who want to burn off some energy.

Room Types

Pop Century only offers a few room types categorized by their location and view.

These rooms are 260 square feet and can accommodate up to four people. These rooms have two double beds or one king-size bed as well as a coffee maker, hair dryer, in-room safe, iron and ironing board, telephone, flat-screen television, refrigerator, and wireless Internet.

Some rooms offer a pool view, which can be louder due to late-night swimmers. There are also preferred rooms closer to the food court and bus stops. Room categories at Pop Century include standard (view of parking lot and far from buses and food court), preferred (near food court and buses but not facing the pool) and preferred pool (near food court and buses with a view of the pool).

Animal Kingdom Resorts

Imagine waking up to an African savannah, Mayan empire, or larger-than-life sport, movie, or music icons. Sound good? Then the resorts near Animal Kingdom are just for you. Although these resorts may be farther away from the other parks, the seclusion they offer may be just the reprieve your family needs from the hustle and bustle of life.

Disney's Animal Kingdom Lodge – Jambo House & Kidani Village

Enjoy your morning coffee on your balcony as you overlook an African savannah with giraffes, zebras, and elephants. That's exactly what Animal Kingdom Lodge allows you to experience. This deluxe resort offers much more, but its theming is unrivaled.

Animal Kingdom Lodge offers bus transportation to all the parks: Magic Kingdom, Epcot, Hollywood Studios, Animal Kingdom, and Disney Springs.

Dining

Between the Jambo House and Kidani Village (deluxe villas), there are many great restaurants to enjoy. (See Chapter 7 for more information.)
Amenities

There are many amenities available for your family to enjoy throughout this resort. Laundry services are available and room service 24/7. Both the Jambo House and Kidani Village offer fitness centers, open 24/7, for those wanting to get in a workout. The Zahanati Fitness Center at the Jambo House also offers a spa and salon for those wanting to be pampered.

Simba's Cubhouse, located in the Jambo House, is available for potty-trained kids aged three to twelve from 4:30 p.m. to midnight. This area with video games, arts and crafts, and movies is a great place to let the kids play while the adults go out.

There are two pools available for guests. The Uzima Pool is located near the Jambo House and includes a waterslide, zero-entry area, hot tubs, and a wading pool for the little ones. The Samawati Pool is near Kidani Village and, although smaller, includes a slide and two hot tubs. A fun addition is the camp area that includes water cannons, puzzles, squirting gardens, and more.

Other recreational activities include an arcade and a community hall area for games, bike rentals, jogging trail, and playground. You can also enjoy your favorite Disney movie under the stars on an inflatable movie screen each evening.

For those wanting a truly exciting experience, there are many animal programs available for you to enjoy. These programs allow an up-close experience.

One caution regarding Animal Kingdom Lodge is its proximity to the parks. With the exception of Animal Kingdom, it can take twenty to forty minutes to get to the other parks using Disney transportation.

Room Types

Both the Jambo House and Kidani Village offer various room types and views. However, a savannah or Arusha view cannot be beat. Seeing animals outside your balcony is a truly amazing experience and well worth the extra cost for an upgraded room view.

Standard rooms are 344 square feet and accommodate up to four people. All rooms have two queen-size beds, one queen bed with a set of bunk beds, or one king bed. Select deluxe rooms can include a daybed and balcony. These rooms offer a bathroom with vanity area. Included in the room is an alarm clock with mp3 player, coffee maker, hair dryer, in-room safe, iron and ironing board, telephone, flat-screen television, refrigerator, and wireless Internet.

Animal Kingdom Lodge also offers concierge level rooms and many types of suites. The one-bedroom suites are 777 square feet and include a bedroom, one-and-a-half baths, and small living area. The two-bedroom suites are similar to the one-bedroom, but include another bedroom. The Royal Kuba Vice-Presidential Suite is 1,619 square feet and includes two bedrooms, two-and-a-half bathrooms, and living area. The Royal Assante Suite is 2,115 square feet and includes two bedrooms, two-and-a-half bathrooms, a dining area, living area, and service kitchen with a microwave.

Disney's Animal Kingdom Villas – Kidani Village

Deluxe villas at Animal Kingdom Lodge include deluxe studios, one-and two-bedroom villas, and a few grand villas. The deluxe studios are 316 square feet and are similar to the rooms at Animal Kingdom Lodge. However, these rooms include a kitchenette with a toaster and microwave. These rooms accommodate up to four guests.

The one-bedroom villas are 710 square feet and include a separate master bedroom and bathroom. Also included is a full-sized kitchen with a larger refrigerator, sink, oven, stove, and microwave as well as plates, flatware, glasses, pots, pans, and more. The master bedroom includes a king-size bed, and the living area includes a queen-size sleeper sofa. This room accommodates up to four guests.

The two-bedroom villas are 1,173 square feet and combine the deluxe studio with the one-bedroom villa. These rooms can accommodate up to nine guests.

There are also a few three-bedroom or grand villas that accommodate up to twelve guests. A few of these villas span over two levels.

Disney's Coronado Springs Resort

Experience southwest Mexico in this moderate resort. From the coral color to the Aztec symbols, you will feel the theming all around you.

Coronado Springs offers bus transportation to all the parks: Magic Kingdom, Epcot, Hollywood Studios, Animal Kingdom, and Disney Springs.

Dining

Coronado Springs includes a counter-service food court and table-service restaurant for families to enjoy two completely different experiences within their resort. (See Chapter 7 for more information.)

Amenities

Since Coronado Springs is also a convention center, it offers more amenities than the other moderate resorts. Included is the La Vida Health Club offering state-of-the-art fitness equipment, massages, facials, and nail treatments. Nearby is a salon for those wishing to get a hair or beauty treatment.

There are three pools available for your family to enjoy. The feature pool includes a waterslide and a dig site for the little archaeologists.

Other recreation opportunities include arcade, bass fishing excursions, a jogging trail, playground, and beach volleyball court.

Room Types

Coronado Springs offers the most room types out of any of the moderate resorts. From standard rooms to suites, there is something available for any family type. The preferred rooms are closer to the food court and bus stops. For those with young children, a preferred room is a must, as this resort is very spread out.

Standard rooms are 300 square feet and can accommodate up to four people. All rooms have two queen-size beds or one king bed. These rooms offer a bathroom with separate vanity area. Included in the room is a coffee maker, hair dryer, in-room safe, iron and ironing board, telephone, flat-screen television, refrigerator, and wireless Internet.

There are a few suites available for those wanting more room. The Junior Suite offers a bedroom, parlor, and two bathrooms. The one-bedroom suite is slightly larger, as it includes an extra bedroom. The Executive Suite includes two bedrooms and two bathrooms.

Disney's All-Star Resorts (Music, Movies, and Sports)

Using bright colors, this resort brings your favorite music, movies, and sports to life in a big way. This value resort will bring out your inner musician, actor, or even athlete.

All-Star Resorts offer bus transportation to all the parks: Magic Kingdom, Epcot, Hollywood Studios, Animal Kingdom and Disney Springs.

Dining

Each section of the All-Star Resorts offers a counter-service food court for your family to enjoy. (See Chapter 7 for more information.)

Amenities

All-Star Resorts offer a few amenities to families. Each section (Sports, Music, and Movies) offers two pools for your family to enjoy. One is larger, and the smaller one us usually slightly quieter.

There is also an arcade for those wanting to enjoy video games. Playground equipment is also available.

Room Types

All-Star Resorts only offer a few room types categorized by their location and view.

These rooms are 260 square feet and can accommodate up to four people. These rooms have two double beds or one king-sized bed and a hair dryer, in-room safe, iron and ironing board, telephone, flat-screen television, refrigerator, and wireless Internet.

Some rooms offer a pool view. There are also preferred rooms, which are closer to the food court and bus stops.

All-Star Music also offers family suites that sleep up to six plus an infant in a crib. These rooms are 560 square feet and include one queen-size bed, a living room with a double-size sleeper sofa, and two twin-sized sleeper chairs, two bathrooms, and a mini-kitchen.

Disney Springs Resorts

Being near to shopping, restaurants, and entertainment is what these resorts offer. With quick access via bus or boat to Disney Springs, you are just minutes away from your favorite shops and restaurants.

Disney's Old Key West Resort

Enjoy the ambiance of the Florida Keys as you relax in the light colors of this Disney Vacation Club resort.

Old Key West offers bus transportation to all the parks: Magic Kingdom, Epcot, Hollywood Studios, Animal Kingdom, and Disney Springs. Ferry boat transportation is also available to Disney Springs.

Dining

Old Key West includes a table- and counter-service restaurant for your family to enjoy. (See Chapter 7 for more information.)

Amenities

Old Key West offers many amenities for your family to enjoy. Get in a workout at the REST Fitness Center which includes fitness equipment, showers, and a sauna. If you are looking for a different way to work out, there are many recreational opportunities. Take your skills to the basketball, volleyball, or tennis courts, or try your hand at classic shuffleboard.

As for rentals, your family can rent watercraft to take on the water or rent bikes to cruise around the property. There are also two arcades for your family to enjoy.

Old Key West has four pools, including the large feature pool with a waterslide, children's area, and hot tub. There are also three smaller pools with a playground and sauna nearby.

The Community Hall is a great place to relax by reading a book or taking on a board game. There is also a movie under the stars, which is a fun way to watch your favorite Disney movies.

Room Types

As a Disney Vacation Club property, this resort offers various types of villas. The views tend to be similar, so focus on the room type that would be best for your family.

Offered are deluxe studios, one- and two-bedroom villas, and a few grand villas. The deluxe studios are 376 square feet with a kitchenette with a toaster and microwave. These rooms accommodate up to four guests.

The one-bedroom villas are 942 square feet and include a separate master suite. Also included is a full-sized kitchen that includes a larger refrigerator, sink, oven, stove, and microwave as well as plates, flatware, glasses, pots, pans, and more for your convenience. The master bedroom includes a king-size bed, and the living area includes a queen-size sleeper sofa. This room accommodates four adult guests.

The two-bedroom villas are 1,333 square feet and offer a master bedroom and bathroom with a second bedroom with two queen beds. Each bedroom has its own bathroom. These rooms can accommodate up to eight guests and are the some of the most spacious accommodations on Disney property.

There are also a few three-bedroom or grand villas that accommodate up to twelve guests. A few of these villas span over two levels.

Disney's Saratoga Springs Resort & Spa

Be transported to a Victorian-style, equestrian-themed resort. This Disney Vacation Club property truly makes you feel you have entered a New York State retreat.

Saratoga Springs offers bus transportation to all the parks: Magic Kingdom, Epcot, Hollywood Studios, Animal Kingdom, and Disney Springs. Ferry boat transportation is also available to Disney Springs.

Dining

Saratoga Springs Resort includes two table-service locations for your family. (See Chapter 7 for more information.)

Amenities

Saratoga Springs offers great amenities for your family to enjoy. One that is sure to please runners is the Senses Spa, which offers massage therapies, facials, body treatments, couples' relaxation packages, and much more. There is also a salon for some extra pampering. Also located at the spa is a fitness center. With cardiovascular equipment and a weight room, there is something for every fitness enthusiast to enjoy.

There are four pools for your family to enjoy. The feature pool offers a waterslide, zero entry, hot tubs, and even a gorgeous water rock display.

Basketball and tennis courts are available, with rentals of bike and other sport equipment. There is also an arcade and playground.

For other family fun, enjoy the Community Hall with games and more. Or enjoy a homemade dinner at the barbeque pavilion for those wanting to grill. You can even watch your favorite Disney movie under the stars.

Room Types

As a Disney Vacation Club property, this resort offers various types of villas. The views tend to be similar, so instead focus on the room type that would be best for your family.

Offered are deluxe studios, one- and two-bedroom villas and a few grand villas. The deluxe studios are 365 square feet. These rooms include a kitchenette with a toaster and microwave. These rooms accommodate up to four guests.

The one-bedroom villas are 714 square feet and include a separate master bedroom and bathroom. Also included is a full-sized kitchen with a larger refrigerator, sink, oven, stove, and microwave as well as plates, flatware, glasses, pots, pans, and more. The master bedroom includes a king-size bed, and the living area includes a queen-size sleeper sofa. This room accommodates up to four guests.

The two-bedroom villas are 1,074 square feet and combine the deluxe studio with the one-bedroom villa. These rooms can accommodate up to eight guests. There are also three-bedroom Treehouse Villas that have a unique theming and are more secluded.

There are also a few three-bedroom or grand villas that accommodate up to twelve guests. A few of these villas span over two levels.

Disney's Port Orleans Resort - Riverside

Nestled by the Sassagoula River, Port Orleans Riverside is full of southern charm. Enjoy the large mansions and cottages of this moderate resort.

Port Orleans Riverside offers bus transportation to all the parks: Magic Kingdom, Epcot, Hollywood Studios, Animal Kingdom, and Disney Springs. Ferry boat transportation is also available to Disney Springs.

Dining

Enjoy a table-service restaurant for a nice meal, or head to the food court for a quick bite before hitting the parks. You can also walk to Port Orleans French Quarter for another meal option. (See Chapter 7 for more information.)

Amenities

There are some unique amenities available at Port Orleans Riverside. One is carriage rides. Enjoy a ride in horse-drawn carriages around this resort. You can also try your hand at fishing in the "fishing hole" with cane poles. Extra cost is involved. The hotel concierge can assist with reservations/rentals.

There are six pools throughout the property, a playground, and an arcade. (Note: Guests of Port Orleans Riverside may be able to use the pool at Port Orleans French Quarter.) For those wanting to experience some recreation, you can rent bikes or watercraft, including Sea Raycers, pedal boats, canoes, and more.

Room Types

Port Orleans Riverside offers some great room types just for families. From water views to royal rooms, there is something for everyone.

Standard rooms are 314 square feet, and some can accommodate up to five people. All rooms have two double beds, two queen-size beds, or a king bed. Some rooms at this resort include two double beds and a small Murphy bed suitable for kids. These rooms offer a bathroom with separate vanity area. Included in the room is a coffee maker, hair dryer, in-room safe, iron and ironing board, telephone, flat-screen television, refrigerator, and wireless Internet.

For those families wanting a truly magical experience, be sure to choose a royal room. Join Princess Tiana in these rooms featuring special details such as royal bedspreads and decorations that are fit for a princess or prince.

Disney's Port Orleans Resort - French Quarter

Be transported to the French Quarter of Louisiana in this moderate resort where every day is a celebration.

Port Orleans French Quarter offers bus transportation to all the parks: Magic Kingdom, Epcot, Hollywood Studios, Animal Kingdom, and Disney Springs. Ferry boat transportation is also available to Disney Springs.

Dining

Port Orleans French Quarter only offers a food court, but you can easily walk to Port Orleans Riverside to enjoy a table-service meal. (See Chapter 7 for more information.)

Amenities

This resort offers the same amenities as Port Orleans Riverside.

Room Types

Port Orleans French Quarter has room types for every family. Enjoy garden, water, and even river views.

Standard rooms are 314 square feet and can accommodate up to four people. All rooms have two queen beds or a king bed. These rooms offer a bathroom with separate vanity area. Included in the room is a coffee maker, hair dryer, in-room safe, iron and ironing board, telephone, flat-screen television, refrigerator, and wireless Internet.

> We really enjoyed Port Orleans French Quarter. It is a close location to start/finish. Very comfortable and quiet resort.
> *Cami, VA*

Running Trails

Even though you are headed to Walt Disney World for a race, you may want to loosen your legs before or after the race. There are many great running trails throughout the resorts. Upon your arrival, ask a cast member or someone at the concierge desk for a map of the running trails. This will give you an idea of the paths you can take.

New Balance has recently partnered with Disney to make these running paths even better. Be on the lookout for signage that will direct you in the various paths you can run.

Most of these trails are under three-mile loops. If you are visiting Walt Disney World during a non-race weekend and need to get in a longer training run, you may need to make multiple loops. Although it is tempting to follow the main roads like the race courses do, this is highly discouraged. There is consistently a lot of traffic, so remember safety first, stay away from the main roads, and stick to the walking paths and running trails.

Here are a few runner favorites:

Boardwalk, Yacht & Beach Club - The path around Crescent Lake along the Boardwalk and even toward Hollywood Studios offers a great option for runners and walkers. Once around Crescent Lake is just under a mile, as is the path to Hollywood Studios and back. Make the loop a few times (or add the loops together) for a longer run or just once for a quick shakeout run. You can also run along Epcot Resorts Boulevard and Buena Vista Drive for a 2.4 mile run.

Fort Wilderness - For those wanting a more trail-like experience, this path offers a nature view. Running around the main part of Fort Wilderness along to Wilderness Lodge is approximately 2.5 miles. Add in some time through the campground, and the run can become even longer if needed.

Saratoga Springs and Disney Springs - This resort is quite expansive, so running throughout the property will create a 1.5 mile loop easily. For a longer run, take the path to Disney Springs. If you're running early in the morning, take advantage of an empty entertainment district. (Keep in mind areas inside Disney Springs may be closed, but there is a sidewalk area outside of the district.)

Grand Floridian and Polynesian Resorts - Beyond running around each property, you can also run along the path between these two resorts. The path between is approximately one mile in length, and you can run along the paths between the buildings to increase the mileage. Running around the buildings of the Polynesian Resort can equal up to 1.5 miles, so there is potential for a nice run.

Art of Animation and Pop Century Resorts - Run around each resort property for approximately a one-mile loop. You can also cross the bridge at Hourglass Lake to explore both resorts and make your run longer.

Port Orleans Riverside and French Quarter - Run along the Sassagoula River from Riverside to the French Quarter (or vice versa) for a mile-long journey. You can also explore the paths around the buildings for an even longer run.

Always exercise caution when running. If it is dark out, be sure that you are wearing illumination-type gear. If it is warm out, be sure to bring along hydration. And always watch your step.

Booking a Room/Package

Once you have selected a resort, there are a few more things to consider. Will you need park tickets? How about the dining plan? If you only need a room, then you should book a room-only reservation. This requires a deposit equivalent to one night's stay. Your final balance is due upon the arrival at your resort.

If you will need park tickets, then you will need to purchase a Magic Your Way Package. This basically combines your accommodations with park tickets (and the dining plan, if you so choose). You can choose base park tickets that allow you to visit one park per day. Packages allow you to purchase a one-day park ticket up to a ten-day park ticket. (Keep in mind, the more days you purchase, the less per day you pay.) Children under the age of three get entrance into the parks at no cost.

For those wishing to visit more than one park per day, you can add a Park Hopper option. This is great for those with older kids or adults. The Park Hopper option adds a flat rate of $64 (plus tax) to any ticket.

If you would like to visit a water park or two during your stay, then adding on the Water Park and More option is a must. For an additional flat rate of $60 (plus tax) per ticket, you get entrance into Typhoon Lagoon, Blizzard Beach, and the ESPN Wide World of Sports Complex, a round of miniature golf at Fantasia Gardens and/or Winter Summerland and a round of golf at Oak Trail. You receive a number of admissions equivalent to the number of days of tickets you purchased. For example, if you purchased five-day tickets with the Water Park and More option, you get five entrances to any of the above locations.

If you choose both the Park Hopper and Water Park and More options, the additional price per ticket is $90 (plus tax).

The next item to consider is the dining plan. The cost varies depending on the plan that you choose, and it can save your family up to 30% on food costs. There are various options, and children aged three to nine will pay a child's rate, while children ten and up are considered adults.

Quick-Service Dining Plan - This plan is best for families on the go. Included are two quick-service meals and one snack per person (ages three and up) per night of stay. Also included is a refillable mug for each person that you can use at your resort's food court or quick-service location.

Dining Plan - This plan is the most popular option. It includes one table-service meal credit, one quick-service meal credit, and one snack per person (ages three and up) per night of stay. This plan also includes one refillable mug per person to use at your resort's food court or quick-service location.

Deluxe Dining Plan - This plan is best for those wanting to experience multiple signature restaurants throughout their stay. Included are three meals (table service or counter service) and two snacks per person (ages three and up) per night of stay, as well as a refillable mug per person to use at your resort's food court or quick-service location.

Premium Plan - This plan includes the Deluxe Dining Plan and adds on some recreation and other extras. Enjoy the following at no additional cost: fishing, golf (at select courses), parasailing, wakeboarding, waterskiing, watercraft rentals, bike rentals, tennis, horseback riding, carriage rides, archery, miniature golf, unlimited use of Children's Activity Centers, select tours, and even tickets to Cirque du Soleil - La Nouba. For a full description of this plan, see **disneyworld.disney.go.com/planning-guides/in-depth-advice/disney-dining-plan**.

Platinum Plan - This is the premiere dining plan. This plan includes all items on the Premium Plan with fewer exclusions. Most tours are available, as well as in-room childcare and use of the Children's Activity Centers. Your family can also experience fireworks cruises, select spa treatments, a PhotoPass CD, the Richard Petty ride-along experience, even dinner at Victoria & Albert's. For families wanting a truly superior experience, this plan is for you. For a full description of this plan, see **disneyworld.disney.go.com/planning-guides/in-depth-advice/disney-dining-plan**.

To book any Magic Your Way Package, a $200 deposit is due at time of booking. The balance is due thirty days prior to arrival.

A common question is how soon you should book your package. The sooner, the better. Your deposit is due at time of booking (ranging from $200 to the equivalent of one night's stay, depending on your package); however, you can cancel up until the thirty day mark with no penalty, as you will get your deposit back. Therefore, it is strongly suggested that you book your room as soon as possible as resorts can quickly sell out (especially host resorts).

Everyone wants a great deal when it comes to vacations, and an Authorized Disney Vacation Planner can make sure that you are getting the best deal for your family.

My Disney Experience

My Disney Experience allows you to customize and personalize your entire vacation. Once you book your Disney resort and package, you can log into My Disney Experience and link your reservation. You can also add any dining reservations you have made. Just make sure your name and email address are the same as the ones in your account.

Along with resort and dining reservations, you will be able to schedule FastPass+ selections prior to your vacation. More information on FastPass+ can be found in Chapter 19.

MagicBands are devices that link your resort room key, park tickets, dining plan meal credits, FastPass+ service, PhotoPass+ media (Memory Maker package), and more. This colorful plastic band goes around your wrist and contains all this important information. There is no need to dig through your backpack or purse for your Key to the World card; it is all available on your wrist. Each family member can choose the color of their band prior to their vacation (orange, red, blue, green, yellow, pink, or grey), and add-ons can be purchased to personalize your MagicBand. The bands are hypoallergenic, though it is always recommended you inquire about any allergies you or your family member may have.

Additional Hotels

While staying at a Walt Disney World resort is the most convenient, there are a few other hotel options to consider. Below is a brief look at these runner-friendly options.

Shades of Green

Are you active duty or retired military? If so, you will qualify for one of the best values on Disney property. Shades of Green is a large resort located directly across the street from Disney's Polynesian Village Resort. Standard rooms are the largest on property at over 500 square feet with suite options available as well. Prices are based upon military rank.

For the larger races weekends (specifically Walt Disney World Marathon Weekend and Princess Half-Marathon Weekend), bus transportation is available to the expo and race starts. This resort also offers a prime viewing location for the Walt Disney World Half-Marathon, Walt Disney World Marathon and Princess Half-Marathon races. Do note that leaving this resort during those races will not be allowed as the main exit for the resort is on the race course. Spectators also may not be able to cross the street to go to the Polynesian while the races are going on.

Guests of this resort do qualify for Extra Magic Hours, however the Disney Dining Plan and MagicBands are not offered. This also means that FastPass+ reservations can be made 30 days prior to arrival. Parking is $15 per night at the resort and theme park parking is not included. However, you can access the monorail by walking to the Polynesian Resort, but do keep in mind that will include some extra walking to your day.

For more information on this resort, visit **http://www.shadesofgreen.org/**.

Swan & Dolphin

Located in between Epcot and Hollywood Studios, the Swan and Dolphin Resorts are another great option for runners. The location is especially convenient for Walt Disney World Marathon and the Wine & Dine Half-Marathon events, as both courses include the Epcot resort area. Race transportation is not available for every race, so be sure to inquire prior to making a reservation.

Although the Swan and Dolphin hotels are located on Walt Disney World property, there are some key differences. The Disney Dining Plan is not available as part of your package and MagicBands will not be included. FastPass+ reservations are made 30 days prior to arrival and there is a fee for parking at the resort. Bus transportation is available to all theme parks and Disney Springs, as well as boat transportation to Epcot and Hollywood Studios.

For more information on these hotels, visit
http://www.swandolphin.com/.

Hilton Bonnet Creek

This resort is located outside of Walt Disney World property, but has recently begun to cater to runDisney runners. Their Marathon Weekends program includes a discounted room rate for all four race weekends in Walt Disney World. Race transportation is provided for the half-marathon and marathon distance races. A pasta dinner is also available as well as complimentary snacks and beverages before those early morning races. There is even a Runner's Concierge ready to assist.

Transportation is available to all theme parks as well as Disney Springs. (This transportation is shared with the Waldorf Astoria Orlando.) There is a parking fee for the resort, as well as a daily resort fee.

For more information on this resort, visit
http://www.hiltonbonnetcreek.com/.

Krista & Megan's Tips

-   Our favorite resorts? For Marathon Weekend and the Princess Half-Marathon Weekend, we love the convenience of the monorail resorts. For the Wine & Dine Half -Marathon, the Epcot resorts (specifically Beach Club and Boardwalk) are within walking distance from the after party.

-   The resorts do undergo (usually much needed) renovation from time to time. You will usually be notified if it will affect your stay in any way, but it never hurts to do a little research on your own as well.

-   Just looking for a place to sleep? Value resorts will do. Want a little more theming, a table-service restaurant, and a little more room? Stay at a moderate resort. Do you want to be close to a park and have access to a gym and the largest rooms? Splurge for a deluxe resort.

-   If you are looking for a lot of space in your room, we suggest the family suites at Art of Animation or the villas at the deluxe villa locations. Both offer separate living areas that are great for those early mornings.

-   Don't overlook the resort restaurants for your meals. Many of the resorts offer fantastic meal options, from food courts to signature dining.

-   Need to change your dining reservations? Did you lose your park map with the hours? Want to add on a day of park tickets? All this and more can be handled by the concierge desk in your resort's lobby. Take advantage as they are very knowledgeable and offer great advice.

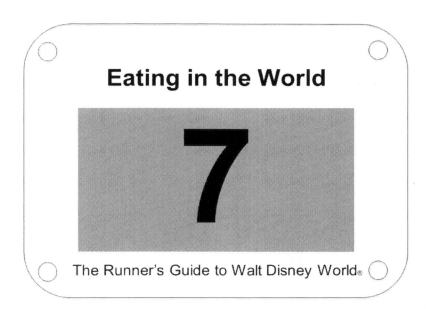

Eating in the World

7

The Runner's Guide to Walt Disney World®

After all your race preparation and training, you may be wondering where and what to eat once you arrive at Walt Disney World. Special post-race celebrations? Food allergies? Intolerances? Pasta? Low-carb? The adults want fine dining, but the kids want chicken fingers? No worries. Novice and experienced athletes alike will not go hungry at Walt Disney World. Runners and their families will find that there is something for everyone during their stay. Whether you are following a strict diet, indulging, or looking for family-friendly dining, Disney has you covered!

Magic Kingdom

Magic Kingdom offers many family-friendly locations for dining. Whether you are enjoying the park prior to the race or as post-race touring, there is something for everyone here.

Based on the surveys from past runDisney participants:

Top 3 Quick-Service Restaurants in Magic Kingdom:
- Be Our Guest (lunch only)
- Tortuga Tavern
- Pecos Bill Cafe

Top 3 Table-Service Restaurants in Magic Kingdom:
- Be Our Guest (dinner only)
- Liberty Tree Tavern
- Crystal Palace

Counter Service

Be Our Guest - Located in Fantasyland, Be Our Guest is a quick-service restaurant during breakfast and lunch hours and a table-service restaurant for dinner. Lunch offerings have a French flair and include items such Croque Monsieur (grilled sandwich of carved ham, Gruyere cheese, and Béchamel sauce) with fries, grilled steak sandwich, and braised pork (coq au vin style) with mashed potatoes and green beans. Healthy offerings include quinoa, shallot and chive salad, and tuna Nicoise salad. For dessert, try the chocolate or fruit cream puff. The kids menu does not contain typical kid fare. So, if you are dining with a picky eater then definitely check out the menu in advance. Offerings include Mickey Meatloaf, mahi mahi, and pasta with tomato sauce.

Casey's Corner - Located on Main Street USA, Casey's serves an all-American fare of hot dogs, fries, and nachos. Popular favorites include the chili cheese dog and the barbecue slaw dog. All specialty hot dogs are served with apples or fries. If you are looking for a meal on the healthier side, you may want to seek out other options.

Columbia Harbor House - Located in Liberty Square across from The Haunted Mansion, Columbia Harbor House is a guest favorite due to the variety of offerings. This nautical-themed restaurant offers hearty sandwiches, soups, and salads as well as fried fish and shrimp baskets. The Anchors Aweigh Sandwich (white tuna with lettuce and tomato served on toasted multigrain bread), grilled salmon with couscous and fresh broccoli, and the Broccoli Peppercorn Salad are popular healthy options. Other popular items include the lobster roll served with chips, New England clam chowder, and fried fish basket. Many entrées allow substituting fries with broccoli or apple slices.

Cosmic Ray's Starlight Café - For those looking for heartier fare, Cosmic Ray's Starlight Café is your "go-to" place in Magic Kingdom. Located in Tomorrowland, across from the Indy Speedway and the Mad Tea Party, this quick-service restaurant provides crowd favorites such as a filling half-pound chicken served with mashed potatoes or the Angus cheeseburger with a "pick your own" toppings bar to create your burger any way you choose. Healthy options are abundant at this location with choices ranging from a veggie burger, turkey sandwich, Greek salad, and rotisserie chicken plate with mashed potatoes and seasonal vegetables. You can choose fries or apple slices with all sandwiches. Parents will be delighted with a turkey sandwich option for kids. However, kids need not be disappointed as there are also Smucker's Uncrustables and chicken nuggets on the menu. Sonny Eclipse, an animatronic lounge singer, performs crowd-friendly music that is out of this world. If you are looking for a quiet place to eat, aim for seating behind the toppings bar.

The Diamond Horseshoe (seasonal) - Since it is only open seasonally during the most crowded times of the year, this restaurant may be closed during most race weekends at Walt Disney World. However, if open, the restaurant serves delicious and healthy options such as a barbecued turkey sandwich, hand-carved pork brisket, tuna salad on a croissant, and a Portobello sandwich, to name a few. Side options are apple slices or potato chips.

The Friar's Nook - This outdoor Quick Service restaurant is located in Fantasyland and is home of several popular gourmet macaroni and cheese options. Selections include Bacon Cheeseburger Mac and Cheese and Mac and Cheese topped with toasted panko bread crumbs. This location has limited hours so if you are looking to carb load then check the Times Guide or the My Disney Experience app for the hours of operation.

Gaston's Tavern - Fantasyland's newest snack location serves up fresh cinnamon rolls and healthy options including hummus and chips and apples with caramel sauce. However, the two stars of this location will be the roasted pork shank and LeFou's Brew, which is a no-sugar-added frozen apple juice with a hint of toasted marshmallow and passion fruit foam.

The Lunching Pad – Located in Tomorrowland under the Tomorrowland Transit Authority PeopleMover, this location is great for a quick meal or snack. While not the healthiest of options, this location does offer tasty treats such as sweet cream cheese pretzels, chips, and specialty hot dog combo meals such as the Philly cheese steak hot dog and the BLT hot dog. Outdoor covered seating provides a great place to people watch in Tomorrowland.

Main Street Bakery - Located on Main Street USA, this popular location often has long lines during breakfast and just before park closing. Breakfast options include the ham and cheddar breakfast sandwich and assorted fresh baked muffins, pastries, and bagels. If you are looking for a late night snack, Main Street Bakery will box up desserts and pastries for you to take back to your resort. Beverages include coffee, cappuccino, or latte as well as bottled soda, water, milk, and juice.

Pecos Bill Tall Tale Inn and Café - Located in Frontierland, this quick-service location is a crowd favorite. Pecos Bill is a large restaurant with tasty options where guests can usually find a seat even on the busiest of days. Seating is divided into different rooms, so if one room is filled then keep going. Popular choices include the barbeque pork sandwich and southwest chicken salad. Pecos Bill is also well known for their Angus cheeseburger and a specialty topping bar to top your burger or salad exactly the way you want it.

Pinocchio Village Haus - Located next to It's a Small World in Fantasyland, Pinocchio Village Haus serves Italian fare such as a variety of flatbreads, spaghetti with meatballs, and a meatball sub sandwich. Healthier options include a Caesar salad with chicken. Kids' meals include mac and cheese, Uncrustables, and pizza. Kids and adults alike will enjoy sitting next to the window overlooking It's a Small World.

Skipper Canteen – Located in Adventureland, this restaurant is scheduled to open in late 2015. To add to the ambiance, the restaurant will be staffed by Jungle Cruise Skippers.

Tomorrowland Terrace Restaurant - Open seasonally for lunch and dinner. Located at the entrance to Tomorrowland, this restaurant may not be open during race weekends. However, if open, the restaurant offers an assortment of selections including a fried chicken sandwich, lobster roll, and a citrus shrimp salad. Bacon cheeseburgers and chicken nuggets are also available. The seating area for this restaurant also serves as the location for the Wishes Dessert Fireworks Party. See Special Celebrations for more information on this event.

Tortuga Tavern (formerly El Pirata Y el Perico) - Located in Adventureland, this restaurant offers Mexican fare including burritos filled with chicken or beef and cilantro rice and black beans, taco salads, and beef nachos. Vegetarian burritos are also available. For kids, quesadillas and peanut butter and jelly sandwiches are available. A topping bar is also available to customize your food to your personal taste.

Table Service

Be Our Guest - Located in Fantasyland, make your reservations early for this location as it is one of the most difficult reservations to get at Walt Disney World. This table-service restaurant offers dinner selections such as sautéed shrimp and scallops, grilled strip steak, and layered ratatouille (vegetarian). Dessert includes a variety of cream puffs (gluten-free offerings available) and cupcakes, which are presented and served tableside.

Cinderella's Royal Table - Dine like royalty at Cinderella's Royal Table inside Cinderella's Castle. Guests choose this location for the atmosphere and the princess interaction, as four princesses rotate through the restaurant tables for autographs and photos during your meal. A new chef and a revamped menu have brought a fresh perspective to this popular location. Breakfast entrées include caramel apple stuffed french toast and grilled filet mignon on a mild chipotle-caramelized onion frittata served with rosemary-lemon roasted potatoes. For lunch and dinner, popular entrées include pan-seared chicken breast served with saffron risotto and a slow-roasted pork loin resting on truffle-farro risotto with a cherry sauce. Popular desserts include a white and dark chocolate glass slipper or lemon sorbet. The meal price includes an 18% gratuity and a photo package of your party with Cinderella.

Liberty Tree Tavern - Located in Liberty Square near the Haunted Mansion, this replica of an eighteenth-century Colonial restaurant serves lunch and dinner influenced by New England dishes. Lunch entrées are ordered from the menu, while dinner selections are served family style. Popular favorites for lunch include the New England clam chowder, New England pot roast with mashed potatoes and garden vegetables, and the Liberty Boys slow-roasted pork sandwich topped with thick slices of bacon, fresh greens, and tomatoes. For lighter fare at lunch, try the Colony Salad with apples, pecans, smoked cheddar, cranberries, and grilled chicken tossed with field greens in a honey-shallot vinaigrette. For dessert during lunch, you won't go wrong with the Ooey Gooey Toffee Cake or Martha Washington's Cake, which is a slice of chocolate cake layered with chocolate icing. During dinner, the Patriot's Platter includes offerings of roasted turkey breast, carved beef and sliced pork with mashed potatoes, seasonal vegetables, herb-bread stuffing, and macaroni and cheese. A mixed greens salad is served prior to the Patriot's Platter. Dessert is Johnny Appleseed's Cake, a tavern-made white cake filled with apples and cranberries topped with ice cream. Dinner is all you care to enjoy.

The Crystal Palace - Guests looking for a classic Disney experience will find one at The Crystal Palace. This popular character dining experience includes a family-friendly buffet with Winnie the Pooh, Tigger, Eeyore, and Piglet. Breakfast and dinner buffet options include traditional American fare. Kid-friendly options include cheese pizza, chicken fingers, and mac and cheese. For dessert, try the self-serve ice cream station or the dessert bar. Located near Casey's Corner, the Crystal Palace is across from Cinderella's Castle.

The Plaza Restaurant - This restaurant serves family favorites in a turn-of-the-twentieth-century classic American restaurant. Crowd favorites include the soup of the day served with either the grilled Reuben or the Plaza Club. The Chicken Strawberry Salad is perfect for those looking for lighter fare, and the meatloaf meal will satisfy those looking for heartier fare. Hand-dipped milkshakes and ice cream floats are among some of fabulous offerings that can top-off your meal. While this restaurant provides a substantial meal, those on the dining plan may wish to use their dining credit at a more expensive restaurant for the best value.

Tony's Town Square - You can't beat the view of Main Street from the outdoor seating at this Italian restaurant. Request a table outside about thirty minutes before a scheduled parade, and you will have one of the prime spots in Magic Kingdom for parade viewing. Indoor décor is themed after Lady and the Tramp. New York strip steak and grilled pork tenderloin are popular selections for dinner and a variety of flatbreads are very popular for lunch. However, for the best in spaghetti with meatballs and baked ziti, try Tony's Town Square. Reservations are required.

Snacks

Throughout Magic Kingdom, there are numerous spots to find tasty snacks. We've chosen to focus on those snacks that are the "best of the best" so that you know where to find these treats. Some items listed below may be excluded from the Disney Dining Plan as a snack credit. Make sure you ask a cast member or look for the Disney Dining Plan icon on the menu.

Aloha Isle - Located in Adventureland, Aloha Isle is famous for the Dole Whip. Dole Whip is a soft-serve frozen treat served in either pineapple, vanilla, or orange. Combination flavors are also available. Dole Whip is served as a frozen treat in a dish or as a pineapple, root beer, or Coke float. On a hot day, there is nothing better than a Dole Whip float to help you get your second wind.

Main Street Confectionery - Located near the park entrance, this old-fashioned candy store has many delicious treats for the young or the young at heart. Create your own combo of M&Ms in your favorite colors or select a chocolate dipped Rice Krispies treat in the shape of Mickey Mouse. Check out the candy counter for a gourmet caramel-dipped apple, fudge in a variety of flavors, or a delicious cupcake or cookie. The delights at this location will satisfy anyone's sweet tooth.

Storybook Treats - Need a snack in Fantasyland? Head to Storybook Treats for a strawberry shortcake sundae or a fudge brownie sundae with hot fudge or caramel topping.

Sleepy Hollow - New menu changes in this Liberty Square location have resulted in some surprising changes at Sleepy Hollow. Previously known for funnel cakes and waffles topped with strawberries and whipped cream or powdered sugar and cinnamon, Sleepy Hollow now includes waffle sandwiches such as the Sweet and Spicy Chicken and the Ham, Prosciutto, and Swiss. However, nothing sounds better for a post-run snack than the Nutella and Fresh Fruit Waffle Sandwich.

Auntie Gravity's Galactic Goodies - Floats, sundaes, and smoothies are the main features at Auntie Gravity's in Tomorrowland. Looking for a lighter treat? All smoothies at this location are made with nonfat yogurt.

Corn Dog and Egg Roll Cart - Located in Adventureland near Swiss Family Robinson Tree House, this cart serves corn dogs and pork and shrimp and vegetable egg rolls.

Turkey Legs - What is a visit to a theme park without a gigantic turkey leg? The main location to find Turkey Legs in Magic Kingdom is at a cart in Frontierland across from Country Bear Jamboree.

Ice Cream Bars and Popcorn - Ice cream bars and popcorn carts are located throughout Magic Kingdom. Crowd favorites include Mickey's Premium Ice Cream Bar dipped in dark chocolate and Mickey's Cookies and Cream Ice Cream Sandwich. Edy's Strawberry Fruit Bar and No Added Sugar Strawberry Bar offer a healthy choice for guilt-free snacking.

Epcot

You can eat your way around the world in Epcot. Try out international cuisine in a fun environment as you experience restaurants from eleven different countries, along with a few American favorites.

Based on the surveys from past runDisney participants:

Top 5 Counter-Service Restaurants in Epcot:
- Sunshine Seasons
- Yorkshire County Fish Shop
- Tangierine Café
- Lotus Blossom Café
- Tutto Gusto Wine Cellar

Top 3 Table-Service Restaurants in Epcot:
- Le Cellier
- Restaurant Marrakesh
- Akershus Royal Banquet Hall

Counter Service

Electric Umbrella - All-American fare is offered at this Future World location. Traditional items such as the Angus bacon cheeseburger with fries and chicken nuggets, along with a veggie Naan-which are offered. Those looking for healthy options may want to head to Sunshine Seasons.

Sunshine Seasons - One of the freshest (and most popular) quick-service restaurants in Epcot. This guest favorite is located in The Land, near Soarin'. Open for breakfast, lunch, and dinner, its popular entrées include Croissant Berry Pudding for breakfast and Panini sandwiches for lunch and dinner. Other healthy options include roasted beets and goat cheese salad and oak-grilled fish or chicken with seasonal vegetables. This location is also very popular due to its many vegetarian options. Numerous options for kids and an expansive pastry counter add to the many reasons to visit this Future World favorite.

Boulangerie Patisserie - Recently renovated, this French quick-service location serves some of the best pastries in Walt Disney World. There are so many fantastic choices that we couldn't begin to mention them all. But anyone looking for a post-race treat will have no trouble finding an indulgence at this location. If you are looking for a meal, Boulangerie Patisserie also sells quick-service meals such as quiches and sandwiches. For dessert, try a chocolate éclair, Napoléon, or caramel soufflé.

Liberty Inn - Located in the American pavilion, guests will find all-American fare in the middle of World Showcase. Typical offerings include burgers and and various salads. Recent additions to this location include a New York strip steak with french fries and broccoli and a grilled chicken BLT sandwich as well as a Red, White and Blue Salad which includes field greens, cranberries, pecans, apples, and blue cheese. Vegetarian offerings are available.

Lotus Blossom Café - Located in China, this quick-service restaurant offers classic Chinese take-out dishes such as shrimp fried rice, orange chicken, and sesame chicken salad. For dessert, try the lychee or caramel ginger ice cream or a mango smoothie.

Sommerfest - Snack on authentic German bratwurst, frankfurters, and beer while listening to live music from restaurants nearby at this covered pavilion in Germany. Delicious desserts and authentic German soft pretzels are great additions to your meal.

Tutto Gusto Wine Cellar - This Italian wine cellar is one of the newest additions to World Showcase in Epcot. Guests looking for a light snack or meal will not be disappointed. Offerings include a selection of Paninis, pastas, and small plates of cheese, vegetables, and authentic Italian meats. Located next to Tutto Italia Restaurant, this small restaurant has limited seating but provides a wonderful authentic Italian atmosphere.

Katsura Grill - Looking for a post-race workout? Guests will climb numerous stairs to get to this quick-service restaurant located in the Japan pavilion. Curries, sushi, and teriyaki combo meals are a few of the highlights. Try the Tonosama Combo, which has teriyaki beef, chicken, and salmon with steamed vegetables and rice. Sake (cold or hot) and Kirin Beer are available in addition to a selection of non-alcoholic beverages.

La Cava del Tequila - A quaint tequila and tapas bar located inside the Mexico pavilion. Stop by for a fantastic margarita or a tasting of a variety of tequila. Tables are reserved for guests ordering tapas, but bar seating is available for those who wish to grab a seat while enjoying a beverage.

La Cantina de San Angel - Who wants Mexican? Head to La Cantina de San Angel for a snack, hearty meal, or anything in between at this lagoon-front cantina. With nachos large enough to share, empanadas, tacos, margaritas, and beer, anyone looking for a Mexican fix will be satisfied with a quick stop here. Outdoor seating near the lagoon is covered. Head indoors if the weather is unfavorable or if you can't find a table outside.

Tangierine Café - Mediterranean favorites such as wraps filled with lamb, chicken, or falafel are popular at this Morocco location. Vegetarians will enjoy the Vegetable Platter, a combination of falafel, couscous salad, hummus, tabouleh, and lentil salad with olives. The Mediterranean Sliders Combo, which is three pita pockets filled with lamb, chicken, falafel, cucumber, and tahini sauce, is also a guest favorite.

Kringla Bakeri Og Kafe - Located in Norway, this is not your average bakery. While this location is popular for authentic pastries such as school bread and Kringla sweet pretzel, guests looking for a hearty sandwich should stop by Kringla Bakeri for a tasty treat such as the ham and apple sandwich, Norwegian Club, or the salmon and egg sandwich. Outdoor seating is covered and plentiful.

Yorkshire County Fish Shop - Serving fish and chips, beer, and nonalcoholic beverages, this popular Epcot location is a great location for a quick meal. Located next to the Rose and Crown Pub in England. Seating is outside and uncovered.

Table Service

Garden Grill - Dine with Chip 'n Dale, Mickey, and Pluto at this rotating restaurant located in The Land in Future World. Rolls, fresh salad, turkey with homemade gravy, sustainable fish, and filet of beef with demi-glace steak butter are served family-style at your table. Sides include mashed potatoes, dressing, and fresh garden vegetables. Dinner is capped off by a delicious seasonal skillet dessert with ice cream. The kids' meal includes a hearty portion of turkey breast, rice pilaf, broccoli, and a fruit cup. This is the only character meal where guests do not have to balance time between running to a buffet and waiting for characters to approach their table, resulting in a more relaxing meal. Garden Grill is open for dinner only.

Coral Reef Restaurant - Located in The Seas in Future World, Coral Reef is not your average seafood restaurant. Guests can dine on baked cheese manicotti with griddled lobster tail, seared mahi mahi with jasmine rice, or grilled New York steak, roasted pork belly, or oven roasted chicken breast for the non-seafood lover. The view is spectacular as guests face the largest inland saltwater environment ever built containing eighty-five different species of tropical fish.

Le Cellier Steakhouse - One of the most popular Epcot locations, Le Cellier is known for great steaks. Located in Canada, this restaurant with limited seating provides an intimate atmosphere for a great meal. Popular entrées include mushroom filet mignon, New York strip, or chicken and waffles all served with delicious sides. Vegetarians will find selections such as the selections of poutine. For a truly unforgettable experience, start your meal with the Canadian cheddar cheese soup and end with the smoking chocolate mousse. Make your reservations 180 days in advance for this popular location.

Nine Dragons Restaurant - Guests can dine on traditional and modern Chinese cuisine in a contemporary Asian setting in China. Cold and hot appetizers such as spicy beef or potstickers are favorites at this World Showcase location. Health-conscious guests will enjoy the Bon-Bon chicken salad or the soup and salad combo. Nine Dragons Family Dinner Set offers soup, entrée, and dessert at a fixed price.

Les Chefs de France - Located in France, this gourmet French restaurant provides a price-fixed menu that will satisfy the hungriest guest. Looking for a lighter meal? Guests can also order a la carte. Soups, fresh fish, short ribs, and beef tenderloin make this restaurant popular with guests. However, the desserts such as fresh strawberry and cream cake served with raspberry sauce and crème brulee make this location a guest favorite. Remy from Ratatouille stops by every table to interact with guests as they dine. Vegetarians can choose from the very popular baked macaroni with Gruyere cheese or vegetable lasagna. Hungry kids will love the cheese puff pastry as an appetizer.

Biergarten - Located in the heart of a German village, this lively restaurant celebrates Oktoberfest all year long. Authentic German cuisine is offered buffet-style where guests eat at long tables. You will be seated with other guests unless your group is large enough to fill the giant tables. However, as the Oompah band performs its twenty-five-minute show every hour and the beer flows, you may soon be singing along with your new friends. Traditional German food is served including sausages, sauerkraut, potatoes, spaetzle, and desserts.

Tutto Italia Ristorante - Looking for a great pre-race carbo-load? Tutto Italia in Italy may just be the place to get your fill. This Italian fine dining location serves classic handmade cuisine that is worthy of a pre-race splurge. Pasta, fish, steak, and chicken are center-stage at this World Showcase location. Side dishes are seasonal, so ask your server about the latest menu updates.

Via Napoli - Southern Italian favorites are offered at this spacious restaurant located at the back of the Italy pavilion. For starters, try Arancini, fried risotto balls filled with mozzarella and topped with meat ragu. Pasta favorites include Lasagna Verde and Spaghetti e Polettine (handcrafted veal meatballs and tomato sauce on a hearty plate of spaghetti). And one of the most popular draws of Via Napoli is the authentic wood-fired pizzas like those found on the streets of Naples. Guests may choose their own toppings or pick a pizza designed by the chef. Either way, you will leave satisfied and happy.

Teppan Edo - Similar to your local Hibachi bar, Teppan Edo is a more authentic version of Japanese cuisine. For example, fried rice is not served at Teppan Edo since it is not considered traditional Japanese cuisine. Located in the Japan Pavilion, entertaining chefs prepare your meal at the grill located at each table. Teppan Edo meal selections include steak, scallops, swordfish, chicken, pork, and vegetables. Vegetables, Udon noodles, and steamed white rice are included. For dessert, choose green tea cheesecake or chocolate ginger cake.

Tokyo Dining - Contemporary Japanese cuisine celebrates modern Tokyo with selections such as tempura chicken and shrimp and scallops served with seasonal vegetables and steamed white rice. Looking for great sushi? Tokyo Dining has some of the best at Walt Disney World. Guests can also choose from a selection of Bento boxes. This location in Japan offers a great view of Illuminations: Reflections of Earth for those who are dining during Epcot's spectacular fireworks show.

Akershus Royal Banquet Hall - Those looking to dine with the princesses will find great food and character interaction at this Epcot location. Located in Norway, the medieval castle-themed restaurant serves authentic Norwegian food such as meats, seafood, salads, and cheeses at breakfast, lunch, and dinner. Less adventurous guests need not worry as traditional American breakfast fare is served family style, and entrées such as chicken, pasta and beef are available during lunch and dinner. Guests receive a picture with Belle with the price of the meal. Four princesses rotate through the tables during dinner greeting guests and posing for pictures.

La Hacienda de San Angel - Traditional Mexican dishes and appetizers are the stars at this waterfront restaurant. For starters, try the Queso Fundido, a delicious appetizer of melted cheese with poblano peppers, chorizo, and flour tortillas. La Hacienda, a mixed grill that serves two and consists of flank steak, chicken chorizo, and vegetables served with beans and fresh salsas is a very popular entrée. This location in Mexico has one of the best views of Illuminations in World Showcase. Make a reservation for 7:30 p.m. and ask for a seat with a view to guarantee a prime spot for viewing the fireworks.

San Angel Inn Restaurante - Inside the Mexico pavilion, this seventeenth-century hacienda-style restaurant features traditional Mexican cuisine where you can watch the boats from Gran Fiesta ride by while you dine. One of the most popular items on the menu is Carne Asada, a New York strip served with cheese enchilada and Mexican rice.

Spice Road Table – located in Morocco, this is the newest restaurant addition to World Showcase. Spice Road Table offers tapas and small plates of authentic Moroccan food. Try a sampling on Fried Calamari followed by Mix Grill Skewers of beef and chicken while enjoying this beautiful location with covered outdoor seating near the water. Kids will enjoy the Watermelon Delight Fruit Cocktail.

Restaurant Marrakesh - North Mediterranean fare is served for lunch and dinner at this Morocco location. While not as exotic as it sounds, Restaurant Marrakesh offers very fresh and healthy entrées such as Mogador Fish Tagine (fish with olives, potatoes, green peppers, and Chermula sauce). Steak or chicken shish kebabs are also excellent choices. Enjoy entertainment from a Moroccan band and belly dancer while you dine. Located in the Morocco Pavilion.

Rose and Crown - English pub cuisine is served at this Tudor-style England location. Open for lunch and dinner, this restaurant offers authentic English favorites such as fish and chips, bangers and mash, and cottage pie. Appetizers include a scotch egg, which is a golden fried hard-boiled egg wrapped in sausage meat with mustard sauce. Healthy choices include the frisée and apple salad with blue cheese crumbles, candied nuts, and cranberry vinaigrette. Outdoor seating provides a great view of Illuminations, although there is limited seating, and only the tables next to the rail will provide an unobstructed view. If you can't get a reservation at Rose and Crown but would like a beer and pub food, try the Rose and Crown Pub. Reservations are not accepted, and they serve a limited menu of British beers and pub grub, including the English Bulldog, a split banger (sausage) served on a roll stuffed with mashed potatoes, chopped bacon, Irish cheddar, and a spiced mustard served with English chips (fries). Keep your cardiologist on speed-dial for this one.

> One of our favorites is Coral Reef. I love the seafood and its awesome atmosphere. The aquarium is amazing and great entertainment while you wait for your food.
>
> *Raegan, IL*

Snacks

There is no place better than Epcot for fabulous snacks at Walt Disney World.

Fountain View - Future World next to the Character Spot. This Future World location used to be known for its ice cream. Recently, this location converted to a Starbucks, which now serves breakfast sandwiches, coffee, lattes, smoothies, and pastries.

Fife and Drum - American Pavilion. This gem serves jumbo turkey legs, Mickey-shaped pretzels, jalapeno-stuffed pretzels, and popcorn.

Funnel Cakes - American Pavilion. The name says it all at this location, with funnel cakes—and that's it—in this gazebo-style stand in America. Try the Pumpkin Spice Funnel Cake offered in the fall.

Crepes des Chefs de France - The American equivalent to the funnel cake, in France you will find the crepes stand. At this location, guests can order a crepe with chocolate, strawberry, sugar, or ice cream. Espresso, cappuccino, French beer, and assorted cold drinks are also offered.

Karamell-Kuche - Those looking for a caramel treat will find exactly what they are looking for in Germany at Karamell-Kuche. Freshly made caramel corn, hand-dipped caramel and chocolate strawberries, caramel apples, dark chocolate caramel with sea salt, and chocolate caramel cupcakes will delight anyone looking for a sweet treat.

Kabuki Café - Look for this stand in Japan, where guests can find a Japanese version of the American snow cone. These unique treats are shaved ice in a variety of fruit flavors and can be topped with sweet milk, strawberry, or cherry. Other unusual treats include green tea or ginger ice cream. Beverages include the standard non-alcoholic drinks as well as Green Tea Matcha Latte, Japanese soda, beer, and hot or cold sake.

Hollywood Studios

Hooray for Hollywood! Eat like a star as you experience fun and unusual restaurants throughout the park. Many guests consider Hollywood Studios to be a "burger and fry" park, but recent menu additions are proving this to be false. Healthy options are now abundant for runners who wish to watch what they eat. Those looking for a sweet treat will find this park offers some of the most delicious and "famous" cupcakes around.

Based on the surveys from past runDisney participants:

Top 3 Counter-Service Restaurants in Hollywood Studios:
- Fairfax Fare
- Starring Rolls
- Rosie's All-American Cafe

Top 3 Table-Service Restaurants in Hollywood Studios:
- '50s Prime Time Cafe
- Sci-Fi Dine-In
- Mama Melrose's

Counter Service

ABC Commissary - Want a blast from the past? Dine at ABC Commissary, and theme songs from your favorite ABC shows will have you singing along to your favorite shows from today and yesterday. Located on Commissary Lane, ABC Commissary has fish baskets, burgers, and chicken sandwiches. Those looking for a lighter option may want to choose the Asian salad or couscous quinoa and arugula salad with salmon or chicken. Kids' picks offer the standard cheeseburgers, chicken nuggets, and turkey sandwiches. All entrées are served with the choice of apple slices or fries.

Backlot Express - Located in Echo Lake between Star Tours and Indiana Jones, Backlot Express is a quick-service restaurant made to look like a prop shop for a movie studio. This quick-service location offers the standard Angus burgers, chicken nuggets, and hot dogs offered at other locations. However, lighter options are available such as the Southwest salad with chicken, grilled turkey and cheese on a multigrain ciabatta, and the grilled vegetable sandwich served on basil asiago bread. Side choices include carrot sticks or fries. Kids' picks have recently expanded to offer more choices including PB&J, grilled vegetable sandwiches, chicken nuggets, and Power Packs (yogurt, apple wedges, carrot sticks, Goldfish crackers, apple-cinnamon snack bar, and a choice of milk or water).

Min and Bill's Dockside Diner – This quick-service outdoor location is great for snacks or a meal on the go. Sandwiches include a frankfurter in a pretzel roll and Italian sausage. All sandwiches are served with chips. This location is a great place to grab a quick meal and while relaxing and people watching on the picnic benches near Echo Lake.

Studio Catering Company - Located at the back of the park near Studio Backlot Tours on the Streets of America, this quick-service location is one of the few places that do not offer burgers. Panini sandwiches including pulled beef brisket, spicy chipotle ranch chicken and turkey and cheese are just a few of the fresh offerings that make this location popular for guest who want to grab a healthy meal on the go. Vegetarian selections include a grilled vegetable sandwich and a Greek salad. Try the marble cheesecake for a delicious dessert.

Toy Story's Pizza Planet – Did someone say pizza? If so, head to Toy Story's Pizza Planet for vegetable, pepperoni, or cheese pizza. A meatball sub and antipasto salad are offered for those who want an alternative option. For a less crowded table, head upstairs or grab a table outside if the weather permits.

Catalina Eddie's - Offers more pizza for guests near Tower of Terror. Limited offerings include pepperoni or cheese pizza, Caesar salad with chicken, and a hot Italian sandwich with Caesar salad.

Fairfax Fare - Open for lunch and dinner. This location provides outdoor seating near Tower of Terror and Catalina Eddie's. Substantial lunch and dinner offerings include a chicken and spare ribs combo with baked beans and coleslaw, barbeque pork sandwich, and gourmet hot dogs (topped with either macaroni and cheese and truffle oil or barbecued pork and coleslaw) with chips. Fairfax Salad offers a healthy option. Kids' offerings include macaroni and cheese, peanut butter and jelly, Power Pack, or turkey sandwich.

Rosie's All-American Café - Options at this location outside Tower of Terror and Rock 'N' Roll Roller Coaster include chicken nuggets, the Angus Onion Straw Cheeseburger, or a vegetable burger. Rosie's is part of the Sunset Ranch Market group of counter-service restaurants, which include Fairfax Fare and Catalina Eddie's. All three restaurants share outdoor seating and allow for large families or groups to experience more variety in one general location.

Starring Rolls - This popular location on Sunset Boulevard is open for breakfast and lunch only. Delicious pastries and gourmet cupcakes are crowd favorites. Specialty sandwiches, which are large enough to share, include a smoked ham sandwich and a turkey focaccia served with fresh fruit and chips. Recent additions include a variety of sushi selections. Kids' offerings include the Kids' Power Pack, a box filled with healthy snacks to keep kids going strong.

Toluca Legs Turkey Company - This is the place to find Turkey Legs at Hollywood Studios. Located near Tower of Terror, covered seating is provided as part of the Sunset Ranch Market group.

Table Service

Sci-Fi Dine-In Theater Restaurant - Atmosphere is the main draw at this popular family-friendly location. And what's not to love? Themed after a 1950s drive-in, complete with convertible cars in which you can dine and sci-fi flicks from the '50s on a big screen, this establishment serves all-American fare. Breakfast is now available at this location. Popular lunch options include burgers and fries. Dessert includes turtle cheesecake and a warm glazed doughnut.

'50s Prime Time - Old-fashioned comfort food circa 1950 is served at this themed restaurant where Mom expects you to eat your green beans and keep your elbows off the table. Your cousins (wait staff) enforce Mom's rules with a dose of good humor. Open for lunch and dinner, hearty favorites include Traditional Meatloaf and Aunt Liz's Golden Fried Chicken. Dad's brownie sundae and old-fashioned milk shakes are the perfect ending to this fabulous meal. Try the Peanut Butter and Jelly Milkshake for a treat that you won't forget when you return home.

Hollywood and Vine - The only character meal in Hollywood Studios, this restaurant located in Echo Lake offers a buffet for breakfast, lunch, and dinner. Characters (Special Agent Oso, Handy Manny, Jake from the Neverland Pirates, and June and Leo from the Little Einsteins) appear at breakfast and lunch only. Breakfast is traditional American breakfast fare such as scrambled eggs, frittatas, Mickey waffles, potatoes, sausage gravy, and biscuits. Lunch and dinner buffets include fresh fish of the day, carved and grilled meats, seasonal vegetables, and a variety of traditional desserts. The Fantasmic! Dinner package is available at dinner only. See Special Celebrations for more information.

The Hollywood Brown Derby - Dine old Hollywood style in this authentic replica of the original Hollywood Brown Derby in California. This upscale dining establishment includes the entrée that made the original restaurant famous: Cobb Salad. White linen tablecloths and wood paneling create an exclusive atmosphere.

Popular entrées include a charred filet of beef glazed with a red wine reduction over white truffle forest mushroom whipped potatoes and grilled salmon with roasted purple cauliflower. Save room for dessert because the Brown Derby Original Grapefruit Cake, which combines layers of yellow cake with fresh grapefruit cream cheese icing, is a unique and refreshing way to end the meal. Kids' options include healthy choices such as tempura fish strips with steamed broccoli and dipping sauce. Fantasmic! Dinner package is available. See Special Celebrations for more information.

Mama Melrose's – Located on the Streets of America, this casual Italian restaurant serves lunch and dinner. Guest favorites include the Oven-Baked Chicken alla Parmigiana and Chicked Campanelle (a pasta tossed in a four-cheese sauce with broccoflower, sun-dried tomatoes, fresh spinach, and sweet onions). Lighter choices include a Grilled Vegetable Flatbread or Seafood Arrabbiata. Desserts at Mama Melrose's provide a fresh twist on Italian classics. For a refreshing treat try the Tiramisu Semifreddo, which is served half-frozen. Kids' meals include an appetizer, entrée, dessert, and drink for a reasonable price. Fantasmic! Dinner Package available. See Special Celebrations for more information.

> At 50s Prime Time, the servers make the meal a lot of fun and the food is great.
>
> *Cristina, NC*

Snacks

Writer's Stop - Located next to Sci-Fi Dine-In, this coffee shop and bookstore is a great place to grab a muffin or pastry and a cup of coffee and relax. Looking for a unique treat? Try the Carrot Cake Cookie.

Starring Rolls - As a previously mentioned in Quick-Service Locations, this restaurant serves hearty sandwiches, but even the most health-conscious person will do a double-take when they spot the cupcakes behind the counter. Well-known favorites include the Butterfinger cupcake and the red velvet cupcake. Other snack options include pastries and muffins.

Snack Carts - Located throughout the park, Hollywood Studios is known for offering the traditional snack options found elsewhere in Walt Disney World. Options that are easy to find include popcorn, pretzels, and ice cream or frozen fruit bars.

Animal Kingdom

Try out Asian and African cuisine at this park. From character meals to eating in the rainforest, every member of your family will find something fun to experience.

Based on the surveys from past runDisney participants:

Top 2 Counter-Service Restaurants in Animal Kingdom:
- Yak & Yeti
- Flame Tree BBQ

Top 2 Table-service Restaurants in Animal Kingdom:
- Tusker House
- Yak & Yeti

Counter Service

Tamu Tamu Refreshments - Grab a snack at this Animal Kingdom location. Various ice cream options are offered, and seating is outdoors and uncovered.

Yak And Yeti Café Window - Located behind Yak and Yeti Local Foods Café in Asia, this walk-up window serves a variety of specialty alcoholic drinks, draft beer, and a ginger chicken salad and Asian chicken sandwich. Non-alcoholic beverages are also available. Seating is outdoors and uncovered.

Yak and Yeti Local Foods Café - Located near the full-service Yak and Yeti Restaurant in Asia, this quick-service restaurant serves Pan-Asian dishes such as a teriyaki beef bowl, honey chicken, and egg rolls. Perfect for a quick snack or light lunch, this location has outdoor seating near Expedition Everest.

Restaurantosaurus - Located in Dinoland USA near The Boneyard, an archeological dig site for kids, Restaurantosaurus offers all-American options for lunch and dinner. Choices include bacon cheeseburgers, mac and cheese hot dogs, grilled chicken sandwiches, black bean burgers, and chicken BLT salads. A choice of fries or apple slices is offered as sides. Kids' offerings include turkey wraps, cheeseburgers, or PB&J.

Flame Tree Barbecue - Located on Discovery Island across from the Tree of Life. Barbecue lovers will delight in the quick-service offerings at Flame Tree Barbecue. Hearty enough to satisfy all appetites with portions large enough to share, guests dining at Flame Tree Barbecue should try the chicken or ribs or get both in a combination platter is. For lighter options, try the smoked chicken salad, fruit plate, or the smoked turkey breast. Seating is outdoor but covered. For a great view, the seating area behind the restaurant is worth the short walk.

Pizzafari - Located on Discovery Island and open for breakfast lunch, and dinner, Pizzafari has beautifully themed dining rooms where guest can enjoy tasty meals such as the breakfast burrito for breakfast and the baked pasta bolognese for lunch or dinner. Pepperoni, cheese, and vegetable pizzas are also offered and served with a Caesar salad. Kids' picks include mac and cheese, turkey sandwiches, and pizza, of course.

Table Service

Tusker House - At Tusker House in Africa, guests can dine with characters such as Mickey, Daisy, Donald, and Goofy during breakfast and lunch. Breakfast includes favorites such as warm banana-cinnamon bread pudding with vanilla sauce and carved rotisserie honey-glazed ham. Guests dining at lunch or dinner will leave satisfied as offering include carved beef top sirloin roast, rotisserie pork loin, and spiced rubbed rotisserie Chicken. Vegetarians will be very happy with the choices at this location, as there are many varieties of salads, vegetable sides, rice, couscous, and pasta on the buffet.

Yak and Yeti Restaurant - Located next to Flight of Wonder, Yak and Yeti offers Asian-fusion specialties such as seared miso salmon and teriyaki mahi mahi. Lo Mein, sweet and sour chicken, and a Kobe beef burger are also popular entrées as guests dine among historic Himalayan artifacts. For dessert, guests should try the fried wontons with vanilla ice cream and honey vanilla drizzle.

Rainforest Café - Located at the park entrance, guests do not need park tickets to eat at this Animal Kingdom location. If you have eaten at a Rainforest Café in your hometown, then this restaurant is identical in theming and menu. For guests who have not dined at Rainforest Café before, the jungle-themed restaurant with simulated thunderstorms and animatronic animals creates an environment that should not be missed. Serving sizes are huge at breakfast, lunch, and dinner. Menu selections include a wide variety of all-American fare, including pasta, burgers, poultry, and vegetarian selections.

Snacks

Animal Kingdom has a wide variety of snack options that are served from carts and stands throughout the park. These are just a few of the highlights:

Harambe Fruit Market - Known for its healthy selections, Harambe offers whole fruits, fruit cups, sliced veggies, trail mix, and soft pretzels including plain, salted, or jalapeno cheese-stuffed pretzel.

Kusafiri Coffee Shop & Bakery - Guests looking for a cup of coffee at Animal Kingdom will want to head to Africa to Kusafiri Coffee Shop & Bakery. A small walk-up window next to Tusker House, Kusafiri sells pastries, cookies, and gourmet cupcakes. Any of the cupcakes piled high with buttercream frosting at this location will satisfy your sweet tooth.

Trilo-Bites - Located on the path from Discovery Island headed to DinoLand, Trilo-Bites sells warm waffles with strawberries and cream and baked apple blossoms with or without ice cream.

Dino-Bite Snacks - Located in DinoLand USA, this location offers hand-scooped ice cream, hot-fudge sundaes, churros, and freshly baked cookies.

Royal Anandapur Tea Company - Specialty coffee drinks and gourmet hot or iced teas are available at this Asia location as you head from Kali River Rapids to Expedition Everest.

Disney Springs

Eat like a rock star, experience a meteor shower, or indulge in an ice cream sundae. Disney Springs offers many restaurants for your family with something that will please everyone!

Based on the surveys from past runDisney participants:

Top 3 Counter-Service Restaurants in Disney Springs:
- Cookes of Dublin
- Ghiradelli Soda Fountain
- Wolfgang Puck Express

Top 3 Table-Service Restaurants in Disney Springs:
- Fulton's Crab House
- Portobello Yacht Club
- Bongo's Cuban Cafe

Counter Service

Cookes of Dublin - Located next to Raglan Road at Disney Springs's Marketplace, Cookes is known for serving up great fish and chips. Cookes also serves Dublin-style pies such as the chicken and field mushroom pie. A few salads are offered as lighter fare, but guests looking for a truly healthy meal should probably head elsewhere in Disney Springs. However, if it's a true indulgence you are seeking then cap off your fish and chips with a Doh-Bar, which is a battered and deep-fried candy bar.

Earl of Sandwich - Looking for a healthy meal? Head to Earl of Sandwich where the lengthy line demonstrates just how popular this eatery is with Disney guests. Serving breakfast, lunch, and dinner, Earl of Sandwich offers hot sandwiches, soups, and salads made to order. Popular items include the Earl's Club and the Full Montagu.

Ghirardelli Soda Fountain & Chocolate Shop - While Ghirardelli's doesn't serve meals, you could easily make a meal out of dessert at this Marketplace location. Ice cream, sundaes, floats, shakes, and chocolate provide guests numerous choices for a tasty indulgence.

The Smokehouse – Located next to House of Blues, this is another option for lunch and dinner. Favorites include the smoked beef brisket, pulled pork sandwich or smoked turkey leg. The kids can even have a mini pulled pork slider of their own.

Vivoli il Gelato – One of the newest additions, Vivoli II Gelato offers fresh and authentic gelato and sorbetto in various flavors. Add a waffle bowl or make it into a milk shake or float. For those needing an extra pick-me-up, specialty coffee is also available.

Wolfgang Puck Express - Come with a big appetite to this quick-service location next to the Christmas Shop. Wolfgang Puck Express is a popular favorite for breakfast, lunch, or dinner. For breakfast, try the tomato, basil and goat cheese omelet or the chocolate chip waffles. For lunch or dinner, try any of the healthy and delicious salads, wood-fired pizzas, or hearty entrées such as bacon-wrapped meatloaf with mashed potatoes, port wine sauce, and crispy onion rings.

Table Service

The Boathouse – New to The Landing, this upscale restaurant is open for lunch and dinner. To make it a truly unique experience, add a ride in one of the amphibicars. Choose from various seafood options as well as steaks.

Fulton's Crab House - Guests looking for fresh seafood should head to Fulton's Crab House where the seafood is flown in daily. Popular entrées include Alaskan king crab claws with red skin potatoes, Maine lobster stuffed with tender gulf shrimp and bay scallops, and Fulton's unforgettable steaks.

Portobello Yacht Club - Located next to Fulton's Crab House, this rustic Italian restaurant serves pizzas from a wood-burning oven. Traditional pastas, salads, appetizers, and desserts round out the menu to create a truly authentic Italian experience. This is a great place to carb up outside of the parks.

Raglan Road Irish Pub & Restaurant - Located in the Marketplace, Raglan Road is an authentic pub where nightly entertainment and a festive atmosphere provide guests with a great experience while enjoying hearty Irish favorites. Try the fish and chips, Keen Eye for the Shepherd's Pie, or Bangers and Booz, but save room for dessert because Ger's Bread and Butter Pudding is a treat like no other.

Rainforest Café - If you have eaten at a Rainforest Café anywhere else, this restaurant is identical in theming and menu. There is another location at Animal Kingdom. For guests who have not dined at Rainforest Café before, the jungle-themed restaurant with simulated thunderstorms and animatronic animals creates an environment that should not be missed. Serving sizes are huge at breakfast, lunch, and dinner. Menu selections include a wide variety of all-American fare including pasta, burgers, poultry, and vegetarian selections.

T-Rex, A Prehistoric Family Adventure - Larger-than-life animatronic dinosaurs and prehistoric creatures invade this Disney Springs restaurant where both the creatures and portions are large. All-American cuisine is offered such as salads, burgers, chicken, and pastas, and there is something on the menu for everyone at this restaurant. Intermittent meteor showers can scare small children.

Bongos Cuban Café - Created by Gloria Estefan, this lively restaurant serves authentic Cuban food in a 1950s Havana nightclub environment. Try Bongos Famous Fried Shredded Beef with white rice, fried plantains, and a black bean cup for dinner or a Cuban club sandwich for a lighter lunch. Vegetarian platters are offered. Kids' menu includes numerous choices including some Cuban selections in addition to the standard kids' fare.

Jock Lindsey's Hanger Bar – Opening in fall 2015, this restaurant is themed around the pilot from the Indiana Jones films. The menu is set to include clever cocktails and appetizers that are easy to share.

Paradiso 37 - Influenced by street foods, Paradiso 37 serves finger-food type cuisine from "Streets of Americas." An extensive menu provides numerous selections of appetizers, salads, burgers, sandwiches, entrées, and desserts.

Planet Hollywood - Open for lunch and dinner, Planet Hollywood serves all-American food in a star-themed restaurant with Hollywood memorabilia. Substantial choices include salads, sandwiches, pastas, chicken, and steak.

Splitsville - Stop by this fantastic new location in Disney Springs for an outstanding meal. Stay for the bowling and games, or just grab a bite to eat! Both will be worth your time, if you wish to enjoy a family-friendly location in Disney Springs. Menu offerings include a variety of pizzas, sushi, sandwiches, appetizers, burgers, and entrées. With an extensive menu, this location is sure to have something for everyone.

Wolfgang Puck Café - Two restaurants exist in one building at Wolfgang Puck Café. Downstairs is a casual restaurant serving lunch and dinner with selections of sandwiches, pastas, salads, and wood-fired pizzas. Upstairs in the dining room, guests will find a more formal restaurant, which is open only for dinner and serves signature entrées such as seared chicken, maple glazed pork chop and a sashimi platter.

House of Blues - A live music club where musicians perform day and night. During lunch or dinner guests can select entrées, appetizers, or sandwiches from an extensive Southern menu. There's plenty of barbeque with the fixin's and plenty of options for vegetarians or health-conscious guests too. On Sunday mornings, a gospel choir performs while a substantial all-you-can eat buffet is served.

Walt Disney World Resorts

Based on the surveys from past runDisney participants:

Top 3 Counter-Service Restaurants at the Walt Disney World resorts:
- Boardwalk Bakery at Boardwalk Inn
- Roaring Forks at Wilderness Lodge
- Landscapes of Flavor at Art of Animation

Top 5 Table-Service Restaurants at the Walt Disney World resorts:
- Jiko at Animal Kingdom Lodge
- California Grill at the Contemporary Resort
- Kona Café at the Polynesian Resort
- Beaches & Cream at the Beach Club
- Sanaa at Animal Kingdom Lodge

Magic Kingdom Resorts

Counter Service

Captain Cook's – Polynesian Resort - This quick-service location is a favorite among many. Located on the main floor of the Great Ceremonial House near the pool area, this restaurant provides unique lunch and dinner offerings including an Aloha pork sandwich, flatbreads, and stir-fry. There is something for everyone! Be sure to get the famous Tonga Toast for breakfast: banana-stuffed sourdough bread battered, deep-fried, and covered in cinnamon sugar. You can even get a Dole Whip for a snack at the Pineapple Lanai located outside and around the corner from the restaurant. Additional seating provides a great place to relax!

Contempo Café – Contemporary Resort - A quick-service restaurant that offers breakfast, lunch, and dinner options. It is located on the fourth floor of the main building. Breakfast is your normal fare: eggs, bacon, waffles, oatmeal, french toast, and even breakfast burritos. Lunch and dinner offerings include sandwiches, salads and, flatbreads. One of the most recent additions to the Contempo Café includes "tossed to order" salads. Other options include numerous a la carte options such as pastries, bagels, and desserts.

Gasparilla Island Grill – Grand Floridian Resort & Spa - This quick-service location offers breakfast, lunch, and dinner. Located near the marina, breakfast fare includes croissants, pancakes, and more. Lunch and dinner include stir-fry, flatbreads, lasagna, salads, and sandwiches. For a healthy option, sandwiches can be accompanied by a cucumber and tomato salad instead of chips. Looking for a quick bite? Don't forget that snacks are available throughout the day.

Roaring Fork – Wilderness Lodge - This quick-service location is open for breakfast, lunch, and dinner. It is located to the left of the lobby near the pool area. Breakfast is the normal fare; lunch and dinner offerings include sandwiches and salads.

Table Service

1900 Park Fare – Grand Floridian Resort & Spa - This is a character restaurant unlike any other. Breakfast and dinner offer different characters, so don't miss out on your favorites. Located on the first floor of the main building near the concierge desk. Join Pooh, Tigger, Mary Poppins, Alice in Wonderland, and the Mad Hatter for a lovely breakfast buffet. You can also enjoy Prince Charming, Cinderella, and the Evil Stepmother and Stepsisters for a dinner buffet that is sure to make you laugh.

Artist Point – Wilderness Lodge - This signature restaurant is a favorite among many. Located just past the lobby on the left, this table-service restaurant offers cedar plank salmon, crispy ranch chicken, and many more excellent options.

California Grill – Contemporary Resort - Located on the fifteenth floor of the Contemporary Resort, guests come for the food and stay for the fireworks! Enjoy flatbreads, sushi, paella, pork tenderloin, and numerous other menu items that are prepared according to season. And don't forget to save room for dessert! Guests on the Disney Dining Plan will need to keep in mind that this signature restaurant is two table-service credits.

Chef Mickey's – Contemporary Resort - A popular character meal for all to enjoy. Join Mickey, Minnie, Donald, Goofy, and Pluto in this buffet-style meal. This restaurant is located on the fourth floor of the main building, next to Contempo Café and is available for breakfast and dinner (lunch seasonally). Be sure to make your reservations at the 180-day mark as this popular restaurant fills up fast.

Citricos – Grand Floridian Resort & Spa - Located on the second floor of the main building, this signature dinner location offers various appetizers including spiced ahi tuna, winter vegetable root soup, and more. The main course ranges from short ribs to grouper. For dessert, from gelato to cheesecake, there is something for everyone. Here's a tip: the madeira-braised short ribs are the same entrée served next door at the famous Victoria and Albert's for a fraction of the price.

Grand Floridian Café – Grand Floridian Resort & Spa - This table-service restaurant located on the first floor of the main building is open for breakfast, lunch, and dinner. Enjoy omelets, eggs benedict, or vanilla-laced French toast for breakfast. How about a strip steak or grilled pork chop for dinner? The Grand Floridian Café offers outstanding dishes. Don't miss this hidden gem!

Hoop Dee Doo Musical Revue – Fort Wilderness Campground - One of the most popular dining shows at Walt Disney World, Hoop Dee Doo Review at Pioneer Hall is a must for many repeat park guests. This old-fashioned dinner show includes a family style all-you-can-eat meal of fried chicken, smoked barbecue pork ribs, mashed potatoes, baked beans, and strawberry shortcake. Unlimited beverages, including beer, wine, and sangria are served. While the food is delicious, the real stars are the performers who sing, dance, and entertain with a comedy act that is fun for the whole family.

Kona Café – Polynesian Resort - This table-service restaurant offers breakfast, lunch, and dinner. Kona Café is located on the second floor of the Great Ceremonial House, between the monorail stop and 'Ohana. For breakfast, there are many great choices, including Tonga Toast, the Big Kahuna (pancakes, french toast, ham, bacon, and eggs), macadamia nut pancakes, a fruit platter, and more. Lunch and dinner offer entrées with a Polynesian twist. Try various sushi, Pan-Asian noodles, or even teriyaki New York strip. Don't forget dessert, which features jasmine tea-infused cheesecake, Kilauea Torte, and a Kona Kone.

Mickey's Backyard Barbeque – Fort Wilderness Campground - A western-style character dance party served up with all-you-can-eat barbecue fixin's is the main draw at Mickey's Backyard Barbeque. Cyclone Sally and Tumbleweed entertain the crowd with rope tricks and country-western dances and songs. Mickey, Minnie, and friends invite kids of all ages to join in on the dance floor. Unlimited food, beverages (including beer and wine for the adults), and ice cream bars leave all guests satisfied. Please note: because Mickey's Backyard Barbeque is performed in an outdoor covered pavilion, it is typically not held in January or February. During the remainder of the year, Mickey's Backyard Barbecue is only performed one or two nights each week. Reservations are required up to 180 days in advance.

Narcoossee's – Grand Floridian Resort & Spa - Another dinner-only location, this restaurant offers views of the Seven Seas Lagoon. It is located next to the ferry boat stop. Many items on this menu are seafood, from mahi mahi to lobster, with several steak and chicken options for variety. This location is very popular for its nighttime view of Wishes. Book a table about an hour prior to Wishes and ask a server for a seat by the window. If window seats aren't available, simply step out on the balcony for a fabulous view.

'Ohana – Polynesian Resort - This table-service restaurant offers two great meals: a character breakfast and a fun family dinner. This restaurant is located on the second floor of the Great Ceremonial

House, opposite the monorail stop. Join Lilo, Stitch, Mickey, and Pluto for a family-style breakfast. Scrambled eggs, ham, fruit, and breakfast breads are brought to your table to enjoy. For dinner, enjoy great wood-fired meats, carved and brought right to your table on skewers. You won't leave hungry at this restaurant where pot stickers, chicken drumsticks, noodles, salad, and the most amazing bread pudding for dessert are served directly to your table.

Spirit of Aloha Luau – Polynesian Resort - This is a dinner show where you are transported to the South Pacific. Enjoy hula, fire, and knife dancers as you enjoy Hawaiian cuisine. This family-style meal includes pineapple-coconut bread, mixed greens, barbequed pork ribs, roasted chicken, rice, vegetables, and even a pineapple bread pudding dessert. Unlimited beverages, including beer, wine, and sangria are served. This meal is outside in an open air area, so it can be cancelled due to weather.

Trail's End Restaurant – Fort Wilderness Campground - This table-service restaurant offers a quality meal for a great price. Breakfast and dinner are buffet. Breakfast offerings include standard fare such as fresh fruit, scrambled eggs, bacon, sausage, biscuits and gravy, and Mickey waffles. Dinner is a hearty buffet of ribs, hand-carved meats, fresh catch of the day, and vegetable sides. The most popular item is the fried chicken. Take-out options include fried chicken meals, pizza, snacks, and dessert. For lunch, stop in for a leisurely meal that you can order off the menu. Popular menu items include fried chicken and waffles and the open-face BLT. For dessert, try the sticky bun sundae.

Victoria & Albert's – Grand Floridian Resort & Spa - This restaurant has earned the AAA Five-Diamond Award for thirteen years and counting. Located on the second floor of the main building, this two-to-two-and-a-half-hour dining experience is like no other. The menu is constantly changing as the world-renowned chefs are always coming up with new items to introduce. For a truly special experience, book the Chef's Table, where the chef creates a menu just for you and explains each dish as it is prepared and served table-side.

The Wave – Contemporary Resort - This contemporary-themed restaurant prepares seasonally inspired meals for breakfast, lunch, and dinner. For breakfast, you can choose the all-you-care-to enjoy buffet or an entrée from an extensive menu that includes healthy options such as an egg white frittata and signature sweet potato pancakes. Lunch and dinner offer numerous hearty and healthy options that are freshly prepared. An extensive menu for kids provides both healthy options as well as kids' favorites such as grilled cheese and cheese pizza.

Whispering Canyon Café – Wilderness Lodge - A table-service restaurant that will leave a smile on everyone's face. Located on the left side of the lobby. Enjoy breakfast, lunch, or dinner with wait staff that will hoot, holler, and maybe even get you in a (wooden) horse race. Breakfast includes omelets, eggs benedict, waffles, and more. For lunch or dinner, choose from meatloaf, maple-glazed trout, or even a skillet of your favorite country fixin's.

Epcot Resorts

Counter Service

Beach Club Marketplace – Beach Club - This is a counter-service location that offers breakfast, lunch, and dinner. It is located to the left of the lobby, near the volleyball courts. Breakfast includes omelets, french toast sticks, and yogurt parfaits. Lunch and dinner offer pizza, sandwiches, and soups.

Boardwalk Bakery – Boardwalk Inn - This counter-service location offers breakfast, lunch, and dinner-type foods. It is located along the Boardwalk, closer to Epcot. For breakfast, choose from croissants, bagels, pastries, and yogurt parfaits. Lunch and dinner include sandwiches and salads. All sandwiches can be made with gluten-free bread. Just ask!

Everything Pop – Pop Century - This food court is open for breakfast, lunch, and dinner and is located near the lobby. Breakfast includes pastries, pancakes, and omelets. For lunch and dinner, you can enjoy salads, sandwiches, chicken nuggets, burgers, pasta, and pizza. Try the famous Tie-Dye Cheesecake for dessert! It's exclusive to Pop Century.

Landscapes of Flavor – Art of Animation - This counter-service food court serves up breakfast, lunch, and dinner. Located near the lobby. Breakfast offerings include smoothies, waffles, french toast, omelets, and more. Lunch and dinner offer international fare as well as pizza, burgers, make-your-own salad or pasta, and a gelato bar for dessert.

Old Port Royale Food Court – Caribbean Beach Resort - This food court offers breakfast, lunch, and dinner options. Centrally located in Old Port Royale. Breakfast is your normal fare of eggs, bacon, french toast, and oatmeal. Lunch and dinner options include sandwiches, salads, meats, burgers, pizza, and pasta.

Table Service

Beaches and Cream – Yacht Club - This little "soda shop" is open for lunch and dinner. It is located just outside the lobby, near the pool. Choose from burgers, hot dogs, subs, sandwiches, and salad. But don't forget about desserts. From milkshakes to sundaes, there is something for everyone, including the kitchen sink. Want to skip the meal and just get ice cream? No problem. There is a separate line for ice cream orders to go.

Big River Grille – Boardwalk Inn - This table-service restaurant offers lunch and dinner. It is located along the Boardwalk, closer to the Swan and Dolphin hotels. Enjoy salads, pasta, steak, ribs, and more.

Cape May Café – Beach Club - Located in the lobby, this table-service restaurant is a character meal for breakfast and a clam bake for dinner. For breakfast, join Mickey, Minnie, Goofy, and Donald in their beach gear at this breakfast buffet. For dinner, enjoy a clam bake with salads, clam chowder, meat, fresh seafood, and dessert.

Captain's Grille – Yacht Club - This table-service location offers breakfast, lunch, and dinner and is located near the lobby. Breakfast includes omelets, waffles, eggs, smoked salmon, and more. For lunch and dinner, enjoy pork chops, pasta, crab legs, and many other offerings.

ESPN Club – Boardwalk Inn - Located along the Boardwalk near Epcot, this is a great table-service restaurant for those who love sports. Lunch and dinner offerings include appetizers, burgers, hot dogs, sandwiches, and more. This is a great place to watch your favorite game.

Flying Fish – Boardwalk Inn - This dinner-only table-service signature restaurant is great for a date night. It is located along the Boardwalk, toward the middle. Entrées include scallops, yellowfin tuna, strip steak, and more. Dining with kids? Flying Fish has some of the best kids' meals at Walt Disney World.

Shutters – Caribbean Beach Resort - This table-service dinner location is located near the Old Port Royale Food Court. Enjoy appetizers such as chicken wings or shrimp fritters. Entrées include ribeye, seared chicken, sustainable fish, and more.

Trattoria al Forno – Boardwalk Inn – This is the newest addition to the Boardwalk area. Open for breakfast and dinner, this table service location is a welcome addition to the Table Service restaurants in the Boardwalk area. Breakfast options include a frittata with roasted red peppers and prosciutto, as well as a granola yogurt parfait. For dinner, runners can carb up with various pizzas and pastas. If you have room, be sure to try the tiramisu or a spoonful of gelato for dessert.

Yachtsman Steakhouse – Yacht Club - This signature table-service restaurant offers dinner only. It is located to the left of the lobby, near the pool area. Selections include many types of steaks, ravioli, beef wellington, and much more. One of the most famous side dishes is truffle macaroni and cheese.

Animal Kingdom Resorts

Counter Service

End Zone (Sports) – All-Star Sports - This food court has breakfast, lunch, and dinner offerings. It is located in Stadium Hall, near the lobby. Breakfast offers omelets, waffles, and even biscuits and gravy. Lunch and dinner include turkey platters, taco salad, burgers, pizza, and more.

Intermission (Music) – All-Star Music - This food court offers similar food to the End Zone. It is located in Melody Hall, near the lobby.

The Mara – Animal Kingdom Lodge - The counter-service location offers breakfast, lunch, and dinner. Located in the Jambo House, near the pool area along the Zebra Trail. Breakfast includes waffles, eggs, quinoa, and even African-inspired offerings. Lunch and dinner include burgers, chicken, pitas, and African stew.

Pepper Market – Coronado Springs - One of the most unusual food courts offers breakfast, lunch, and dinner. It is centrally located near El Centro or the lobby area. Breakfast includes omelets, skillets, burritos, and more. Lunch and dinner include quesadillas, sandwiches, stir fry, and salads.

World Premiere (Movies) – All-Star Movies - This food court is similar to the End Zone and Intermission. It is located near the lobby, in Cinema Hall.

Table Service

Boma – Animal Kingdom Lodge - This table-service buffet-style restaurant is available for breakfast and dinner and is located on the lower level of Jambo House. For breakfast, enjoy a wide selection of your favorite breakfast foods, along with African-inspired options. Dinner offers everything from curried coconut seafood soup to roasted salmon.

Jiko – Animal Kingdom Lodge - This signature restaurant (two table service credits on the Disney dining plan) offers bold flavors for dinner. It is located near the lobby in Jambo House, next to Boma. Enjoy maize-crusted monkfish, lam or oak-grilled filet mignon.

Maya Grill – Coronado Springs - This table-service restaurant is open for dinner. It is located near the Pepper Market. Options include duck confit, tex mex platters and a fresh catch of the day.

Sanaa – Animal Kingdom Lodge - Open for lunch and dinner, this table-service restaurant offers views of the African savannah. It is located in Kidani Village, near the lobby. You can choose to enjoy samplers of many types of meat and vegetables served with rice. You can also enjoy fish, strip steak, or chicken. Book this restaurant before sunset for a great view of animals on the savannah.

Disney Springs Resorts

Counter Service

Good's Food To Go – Old Key West - This is a counter service area for a quick breakfast, lunch, or dinner. Located in the Hospitality House, near the lobby. Breakfast includes croissant sandwiches and cereal. Lunch and dinner offer burgers, sandwiches, and salads.

Riverside Mill – Port Orleans Riverside - This is a counter-service food court open for breakfast, lunch, and dinner. It is located in the main lobby area. Breakfast includes french toast, create-your-own omelets, waffles, and more. For lunch and dinner, enjoy a fish basket, hamburger, pizza, pasta, and more.

Sassagoula – Port Orleans French Quarter - This counter-service food court offers breakfast, lunch, and dinner. It is located in the main lobby area. Breakfast includes omelets, biscuits and gravy, waffles, and, perhaps the most popular, beignets. Lunch and dinner offer pizza, sandwiches, po'boys, salads, and more.

Table Service

Artist's Palette – Saratoga Springs - This table-service restaurant located in the Carriage House is a cozy place for your family to eat breakfast, lunch, and dinner. Breakfast includes flatbreads, sandwiches, waffles, and more. Lunch and dinner offer Panini sandwiches, salads, and flatbreads.

Boatright's – Port Orleans Riverside - This dinner-only table-service restaurant is actually a restored boat workshop. It is located in the main lobby. Entrées include jambalaya, pork chop, catfish, and other Louisiana Bayou favorites.

Olivia's Café – Old Key West - Open for breakfast, lunch, and dinner, this casual table-service restaurant is a great on-property option located in the Hospitality House. Breakfast includes pancakes, poached eggs, and more. Lunch and dinner offerings include pork chop, meatloaf, fish, and salads.

Turf Club Bar & Grill – Saratoga Springs - Located in the Carriage House, near the Artist's Palette, this table-service restaurant serves lunch and dinner. Entrées include tuna, salmon salad, pasta with shrimp, and more. This all-American restaurant is a great hidden gem. If you are having trouble finding a reservation at other locations, give Turf Club Bar & Grill a try.

Pre-Race Meal Recommendations

Fueling up before the race is one of the best things runners can do to ensure they have plenty of energy. What type of pre-race meal should you enjoy? The best bet is to stick with foods similar to those you ate prior to your long training runs at home. Night races pose a different challenge for the pre-race meal. Practice several long night runs at home and see what types of foods work best. Whatever you decide to eat, rest assured Walt Disney World will have a restaurant to fit your needs.

Here are some great options to consider.

Carb-Loading Options:
- Via Napoli in Epcot
- Tutto Italia in Epcot
- Tony's Town Square in Magic Kingdom
- Mama Melrose's in Disney's Hollywood Studios
- Portobello in Disney Springs
- Everything Pop! at Pop Century Food Court (Italian station)
- Landscape of Flavors Food Court at Art of Animation (make-your-own pasta bar)

Lighter Options:
- The Wave at the Contemporary Resort
- Coral Reef at Epcot
- The Plaza Restaurant in Magic Kingdom
- Sunshine Seasons in Epcot
- Kona Café at the Polynesian Resort

Race Morning Suggestions

When you get up in the middle of the night to run a race, where do you eat? If you are staying at a host resort, the quick-service locations open at 3 a.m. for the morning races. This allows you to grab some food before heading on the bus. A menu isn't set, but carbs and fruit will definitely be included. You have a couple of other options. If you typically eat a pre-run meal at home that would be considered portable (such as bagels and peanut butter, energy bars, etc.) toss some of these in your suitcase. Another option is to shop the food court the night before. Take some yogurt, fresh fruit such as bananas and apples, or granola bars back to your room to eat before you leave the resort.

One recommendation is to take something to eat with you to the race. If you leave your resort at 3:30 a.m. and don't start your race until 5:45 a.m. or later, then you may be hungry again. One important part to remember is you are just starting to run around 5:45 a.m., so you want to make sure you aren't running on an empty stomach. A breakfast consumed at 3:30 a.m. may be long gone by the time a runner reaches Cinderella's castle at 6:30-7 a.m. (and this is just the halfway point for two of Disney's races). Fuel up before leaving the resort, and have a light snack in the corral. You won't be sorry.

> Be sure to check out the food options early and make reservations for the night before your race(s). I would also go a couple days before the race to the food court/quick service area to pick up a couple bananas just in case they run out.
> *Pam, NC*

Celebration Meal Suggestions

You did it! The race is over and now it's time to celebrate. A post-race celebration meal is a great way to cap off your accomplishment. From the ultimate dining experience at Victoria and Albert's to a fun and festive meal at a food court, Disney has your celebration covered. Most runners will wear their race t-shirt from the expo and race medal or medals to their post-race celebration. And why not? You've earned it! Don't forget to make reservations. Some restaurants fill quickly at 180 days pre-race, making reservations for popular locations a necessity.

Here are some great options for you to consider.

At Magic Kingdom:
- Dine with royalty at Cinderella's Royal Table.
- Enjoy the Fireworks Dessert Party at Tomorrowland Terrace (dessert only).
- Experience great hospitality at Be Our Guest.

At Epcot:

- Celebrate German-style and sing along with a German Polka Band and plenty of beer at Biergarten.
- Dine with Mickey and friends at the Garden Grill.
- Le Cellier offers one of the best steaks at Walt Disney World with other fabulous menu options.
- Enjoy some post-race carbs at Tutto Gusto or Via Napoli.
- Have a celebratory drink (or two) at any country in World Showcase.

At Hollywood Studios:

- Enjoy great atmosphere and food at the upscale Hollywood Brown Derby.
- Book a Fantasmic! dinner package. Enjoy a great meal at Mama Melrose's, Hollywood and Vine, or Hollywood Brown Derby followed by reserved seating for Fantasmic!

At Disney Springs:

- Dine on the freshest seafood around at Fulton's.
- Experience fantastic Irish entertainment and food at Raglan Road Irish Pub.
- Take a ride on an amphibicar along with dinner at The Boathouse.

At the resorts:

- Book a Fireworks Cruise at Magic Kingdom or Epcot and enjoy Wishes or Illuminations from a private boat on the water.
- Celebrate with the Fab 5 (Mickey, Minnie, Pluto, Goofy, and Donald) at Chef Mickey at the Contemporary.
- Try the Yachtsman for a fantastic steak dinner in an upscale setting at the Yacht Club.
- Luau with the best at The Spirit of Aloha Dinner Show at the Polynesian.
- Laugh until it hurts at the Hoop Dee Doo Review at Ft. Wilderness.

- Watch the fireworks while you dine at California Grill (Contemporary) or Narcoossee's (Grand Floridian).
- And, for the ultimate in dining experiences, try Victoria and Albert's, an experience that is truly fit for royalty!

Whatever way you choose to celebrate, rest assured that you will have a memorable experience to cap off your hard work.

Advanced Dining Reservations

For any table-service meal at Walt Disney World, it is highly recommended that you make advance dining reservations. It is very rare that you can walk up to a restaurant and get a reservation for that day or even that weekend.

Advance dining reservations are available 180 days prior to your arrival. Call 1-407-WDW-DINE or go to **disneyworld.disney.go.com/reservations/dining** (be sure to sign into your My Disney Experience account first). You can make reservations for your entire stay on the 180-day mark as long as you are staying at a Disney resort. Dining reservations are available up to fifteen minutes prior or twenty minutes after your reserved time, so be sure to make your reservations accordingly, giving your party enough time to travel to the restaurant.

There are a several restaurants that fill up quickly, including Cinderella's Royal Table, 'Ohana, Chef Mickey's, Le Cellier, Be Our Guest, and all dinner shows. If you are interested in any of these popular restaurants, be sure to call in on the 180-day mark at 7 a.m. EST.

Krista & Megan's Tips

- For any table-service restaurant, make reservations! These reservations can be made 180 days from your arrival date and are necessary for most restaurants. You *will* be turned away if you do not have a reservation and there is no room. (Note: No reservations are needed for quick-service locations.)

- All Walt Disney World restaurants will accommodate dietary restrictions. When making your table-service reservations, explain your allergy or dietary needs. The chef will come to your table and go over what is safe for you to eat or will make you your own dish. At quick-service locations, ask for a manager. They will ensure your food is safe!

- When choosing your post-race meal, it may be wise to make it close to your resort. Your legs may be sore, and a long walk may not be in the cards! (Or allow enough time to shuffle your way to the restaurant.)

- Don't overlook the Walt Disney World Resort hotel restaurants! We have found a few of our favorite meals to be inside the Walt Disney World Resort hotels.

- Character meals are a great way to get photos with your new race medal!

- Didn't get the reservation you wanted? Keep checking, especially the day before! Cancellations are made 24 hours in advance.

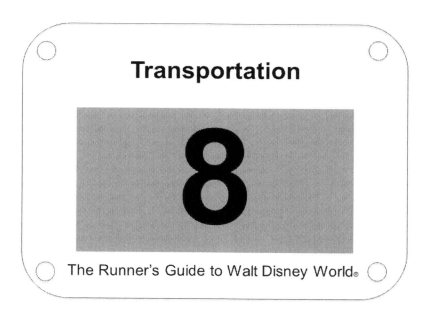

Transportation

8

The Runner's Guide to Walt Disney World®

Whether you are flying or driving, you will be able to get around the Walt Disney World Resort with ease. Staying on Disney property gives you the ability to have the transportation handled for you.

Getting to the World

Magical Express

If you are flying into Orlando International Airport (MCO), Disney offers a great complimentary service to those staying on Disney property. Disney's Magical Express will take you directly from the airport to your resort and back to the airport on your departure day. And even better, they will handle your luggage for you.

It is really simple. If you are taking advantage of Disney's Magical Express, prior to your vacation you will receive yellow tags. Attach these to any checked baggage on one of the handles. By doing so, you can bypass baggage claim upon your arrival in Orlando.

When you arrive in Orlando, go to the B side of the terminal down to Level 1. Disney's Magical Express is located at the end of Level 1 (past the car rental locations). Be sure to have your Disney booklet or MagicBands handy as your Magical Express code is inside. Hand this to the first Disney Cast Member you see, and they will direct you to the correct line for your resort. Forgot your Disney booklet or packed your MagicBands? No worries. Just go to the Magical Express desk and give your name. They will print off your paperwork.

Then sit back, relax, and enjoy the movie as you head to your resort. The trip can take up to an hour depending on how many resorts your bus stops at, so plan accordingly. Your luggage will magically appear in your room up to three hours later. Since it does take a while for your luggage to come to your room, make sure that anything you will need right away is in your carry-on. A change of clothes, swimsuit, medications, your MagicBands and tennis shoes (for heading straight to the parks) may be good things to pack in your carry-on.

The day before your departure, a Magical Express envelope will be in your room. Inside is the time that you need to be at the Magical Express bus stop to head back to the airport. If you have not received it the day prior to your departure, please contact Magical Express at **866-599-0951** for your departure time.

If you would like, you can check your bags at the resort's airline desk so that you don't need to lug your bags through the airport. This service is available for the following airlines: AirTran Airways, Alaska Airlines, American Airlines, Delta Air Lines, JetBlue Airways, Southwest Airlines, United Airlines, and US Airways. Be sure to check your bags prior to your Magical Express departure. If your airline is not listed, you can still utilize Magical Express, but you will need to carry your own bags to the Magical Express bus and check them at the airport upon arrival.

Renting a Car

Although certainly not required, some guests may want to rent their own car upon arrival at the airport. All major car rental companies are located at Orlando International Airport. Once you've picked up the keys to your car, the rental company will provide directions and maps to your Disney resort. It's about a twenty-five-minute drive to Walt Disney World from Orlando International. While Walt Disney World Resort has a comprehensive transportation system, guests who choose to dine at different resorts throughout Walt Disney World will find a rental car to be the most convenient option. Buses from the resorts only transport guests to theme parks. Therefore, guests who need to go from one resort to another resort must first go to a theme park to switch buses. This method of transportation can be extremely time consuming if you find yourself traveling from one resort to another numerous times during your vacation.

Town Car

Town car services are very convenient, reasonably affordable, and an extremely comfortable ride. For round-trip service from the airport to your resort and back, you can expect to pay an average of $120 plus tip. This rate is comparable to a taxi cab fare to Walt Disney World Resort with less hassle. Several added benefits you can expect with a town car service include a driver at baggage claim to meet you when your plane arrives. The driver will assist you with your bags, and you will quickly be on your way to your resort. Town cars tend to be late-model sedans (Lincoln) or SUVs (Tahoe, Suburban) that are comfortable, clean, and spacious. Trunks will easily accommodate numerous pieces of luggage and even golf clubs. Call ahead if you need a car seat provided. Town car services should be scheduled at least twenty-four hours in advance to guarantee availability and pick-up time. Recommended town car company options include Tiffany Town Car Service **tiffanytowncars.com**.

Driving Your Own Car

Perhaps you decide to forego the airlines and drive to Walt Disney World Resort in your own car. If so, you may find that you use your car often or you may park it for the week and chose to rely on resort transportation. Either way, there is plenty of parking available at all of the Disney resorts. Valet parking is available for a fee (around $16 per night) at deluxe resorts. However, self-parking is free at all resorts for resort guests. You will be provided with a parking pass during your resort check-in. Should you choose to drive to the theme parks, your resort parking pass will also allow you to park for free at any theme park throughout your stay.

Cabs

Cabs are available at Orlando International Airport and can transport four to eight individuals, depending upon size. While cab fare is determined by distance and time, you can expect to pay an average of $60 plus tip from the airport to Walt Disney World Resort.

Expo Transportation

If you are looking at a map of Walt Disney World, you may notice that many resorts are very close in proximity to Wide World of Sports where the race expo is held. Being active, you may think that it is a good idea to take a pre-race stroll over to the race expo. However, there are no walking paths, sidewalks, or even service lanes on the roads leading to Wide World of Sports. For safety reasons, participants should not attempt to walk to the race expo held at Wide World of Sports. Fortunately, there are options available for getting to the expo.

Expo Buses

If you are staying at a host resort, motor coach transportation is provided to and from the expo. Head to the front entrance of your resort where there will be signs for the runDisney Expo buses. These buses usually depart every twenty minutes or so.

Once at the expo, pay attention to where your resort's bus is parked. (There are usually signs outside on the parking area and on the bus.) The walk to the expo area is quite a hike, so be sure to wear comfortable shoes and take it easy so you don't wear out your legs before race day. When you have shopped until you dropped, head back to the parking area and follow the signs to your resort's bus. They will take you to your resort where you can drop off your goodies, then head to a park—or the pool.

Cabs

For convenience, cabs are available at your resort to transport you directly to the expo entrance. Fares vary, depending on the distance of your resort to Disney's Wide World of Sports. A reasonable estimate would be $10 plus tip each way for those resorts closest to Wide World of Sports such as Pop Century and Art of Animation and between $15-$25 plus tip for most other resorts. There are cabs at the expo exit, so you can get back to your resort with ease. Keep in mind that traffic congestion during peak times will cause an increase in fares.

Driving Your Own Car

Want to drive your own car to the race expo? If so, you won't have trouble finding a place to park, although once parked you may have a long walk from your car to the expo entrance. Ask for a map of Walt Disney World Resort at check-in, and you can head over to the expo at ESPN Wide World of Sports at your leisure without waiting for bus transportation.

Pre- and Post-Race Transportation

Wondering how you are going to get to a race that starts and ends in different locations? Or one that begins at 5:30 a.m.? Or how you will get to your race while your family is elsewhere? Don't worry! Disney has you covered.

Race Buses

If you are staying at a host resort, the buses that will transport you to the race will be located in the same spot as you took them to the expo: the front entrance. Buses will start to transport runners approximately 2.5 hours prior to the race start and run for approximately one hour. Spectators may also take the bus to the race start, though priority is given to the runners. (It is highly recommended that spectators take the earlier buses to ensure you are able to see your runner along the course or at the finish, especially for the morning races.)

For Walt Disney World Marathon Weekend and Princess Half Marathon Weekend, event transportation is also included for Shades of Green as well as Walt Disney World Swan and Dolphin. As a reminder, walking to the starting corrals from your resort is not allowed and may result in disqualification.

Depending on the race, you may have to walk a ways to get to the actual start line. Keep this in mind. After being dropped off, you can check your bag, use the bathrooms, stretch, and warm up.

Once your race is over, you can use the bus transportation back to your resort. In the family reunion area, you will see a line of buses. Find the bus with your resort's name on it, and you can head back to your resort in the comfort of a temperature-controlled bus.

> Don't stress if it's your first runDisney event. There are lots of signs in the lobby to help you get from your resort to the expo/races.
>
> *Meghan, VA*

Disney Park Transportation

Since most of the larger morning races end after the park opens, you can use Disney park transportation after the race as well. Head back to your resort, or keep moving and head to another Disney park. Most races end in Epcot, which means you can even ride Disney's highway in the sky, the monorail. Expect long lines for resort buses at times. During inclement weather, race participants and spectators may overwhelm the bus system to create long waits.

Cabs

If you don't want to rely on bus transportation, then plan on carrying some cash with you during the race. While secure, leaving cash in your bag check is not recommended as bags are transported and handled by many individuals, and anything can happen. Cabs are located near park transportation and can be very convenient if you are in a hurry to change and get to the parks and in the case of inclement weather or post-run illness. Most runners will not need to take a cab post-run, but it's better to be safe. Tucking some money away pre-race will keep you safe, not sorry.

Driving Your Own Car

Want to drive your own car to the race but wondering if the roads will be blocked? Good news. Yes, you can drive your own car, and, if you leave your resort with plenty of time to spare, driving to the race is possible. Parking is free for resort guests or anyone entering the parks prior to the park's opening.

In most cases, you will want to leave your car at the race finish. If you are running in the Wine & Dine Half-Marathon, you will want to leave your car at Epcot after 7 p.m. and board a race shuttle to ESPN Wide World of Sports for the start.

In the case of early morning races that start at Epcot, you should plan to leave your resort by 3:45 a.m. at the latest. One advantage of driving to the race is that you can stay in your car for quite a while prior to heading to the start line. If it's cold, then you will have a toasty place to have breakfast while waiting for the other runners to arrive. All runners should be in their assigned corral at least forty-five minutes prior to the race's start. If you choose to drive your own car, it's important to note that you should not put your car keys in your checked bag. While rare, checked bags have been known to go missing. Make sure you have a secure place to put your keys while you run!

Park Transportation

In addition to race shuttles and motor coach transportation, Walt Disney World offers an extensive transportation system that will take you anywhere you want to go. Some methods of transportation are more convenient than others, but ultimately Disney transportation can get you there.

Park Shuttles

Park shuttles are the most common way to get around Walt Disney World. Buses depart approximately every fifteen minutes throughout the day until two hours after park closing. Upon checking into your resort, you will receive a resort map that shows where the bus stop is located at your resort. The destination of each bus will appear on the front. However, it is likely that your bus may make more than one stop prior to arriving at its destination. When you are ready to return to your resort, bus stops are located at the exit of each park and throughout Disney Springs. Check the signs for your resort bus stop number, and you will be heading back to your resort in no time.

There are a few things to note about buses. Strollers are allowed on board, but you must be able to fold your stroller and carry it on the bus. If there are not enough seats on board the bus, you will be allowed to stand. All buses are handicapped accessible and usually allow for two or three scooters or wheelchairs to be transported at one time. Bus drivers will assist with loading and unloading of scooters and wheelchairs.

Your Own Car

Just as driving your own car to the race start can be convenient, so can driving to a theme park or Disney Springs. The main advantage to driving is not having to wait for a bus or make numerous stops along the way to your destination. If the line for your resort is lengthy at the end of the evening, you can depart for your resort quickly by heading to your car. Parking is free for the length of your stay at the Walt Disney World Resort. It is usually faster to drive to Disney Springs and to all parks with the exception of Magic Kingdom. Magic Kingdom requires parking at the Transportation and Ticket Center, where guests then board the monorail or ferry to get to Magic Kingdom.

Monorail

Disney's most famous mode of transportation is the monorail, which provides transportation from Contemporary, Polynesian, and Grand Floridian Resorts to Magic Kingdom. You may also take the monorail to Epcot by transferring to the Epcot monorail at the Transportation and Ticket Center. Anyone can ride the monorail at Walt Disney World Resort. Those wishing to park-hop between Magic Kingdom and Epcot will find the monorail to be the fastest and most effective way of getting from one park to another. Strollers are allowed and do not need to be folded. The monorail is also handicapped-accessible. Wheelchairs and scooters are easily loaded and unloaded from the monorail. Cast members will assist guests with this process.

Boat

Boat transportation is located throughout Walt Disney World resort. Ferries take guests from Transportation and Ticket Center to Magic Kingdom. Boat service also runs between Polynesian, Grand Floridian, and Magic Kingdom. Wilderness Lodge and Ft. Wilderness guests can also enjoy a boat ride to Magic Kingdom. This route usually makes a stop at the Contemporary Resort too. If you are staying at Yacht Club, Beach Club, or Boardwalk Inn, you can take a boat to Epcot or Hollywood Studios. Guests at Old Key West, Saratoga Springs, Port Orleans Riverside, and Port Orleans French Quarter all can enjoy boat access to Disney Springs, which is one of the most beautiful and relaxing boat rides at Walt Disney World. Boats are wheelchair and stroller accessible. Strollers on smaller boats may need to be folded.

Cab

Guests who want to make an early dining reservation or park entry may wish to take a cab to the park. If so, cabs are readily available near the main entrance to each resort. Bell services will assist you by calling a cab to come pick you up. Upon exiting the park, you will see a cab line near resort bus transportation. If you want to take a cab to Magic Kingdom for park entry, you should ask the cab to drop you off at the Contemporary Hotel and then take a quick walk over to Magic Kingdom.

Krista & Megan's Tips

- Staying on Disney property at a host resort is the best option for a race weekend. All transportation is provided, which brings much peace of mind!

- Always err on the side of caution and allow yourself more time than you plan to need. It is better to arrive to a race early than be running into the corral at the last minute!

- You must pick up your own race packet. Therefore, if you have a later flight the day prior to the race, it would be best to take a cab or town car from the airport to your resort (or even directly to the expo). This will save quite a bit of time, ensuring you get your race packet before the expo closes!

- If you are using Magical Express, keep in mind that you will be picked up three hours before your flight departure to head back to the airport. You may want to schedule a later flight to avoid another early wake up call.

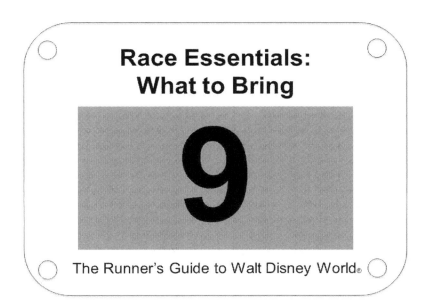

Race Essentials: What to Bring

9

The Runner's Guide to Walt Disney World®

Packing for a vacation is one thing. Packing for a race is another. Not only do you need to make sure you have the essentials packed for touring the parks with your family (plus all of their essentials), you must also make sure that you have everything you will need for race day. Below are some suggestions and reminders on items to pack to ensure your race is successful and fun, along with packing lists in the appendix.

Packing for Vacation

When packing for a trip to Walt Disney World, there are some essentials to remember: a camera, your wallet, and comfortable shoes. Beyond these essentials, you must remember that Florida weather can change from day to day. Here are some tips and tricks to make sure your packing goes smoothly before you leave.

The first thing is to check the weather. Take a look at the extended forecast to get an idea of what to expect, and then pack a few extras. For the January races, it may be cold, but the next day it may be hot, so you need to prepare for all types of weather. For the November race, you may need to prepare for rain. Checking the forecast will allow you to know whether you need to bring four sweatshirts or just one.

You will want to bring comfortable clothes for the parks. A lot of ground is covered when walking around the theme parks (some pedometers have measured over 10 miles), so make sure you feel at ease. Depending on the weather, you will want to bring tank tops, t-shirts, shorts, jeans, sweatshirts, a light jacket, swimsuit, and pajamas. Bring a dressier outfit if you wish to be fancy for dinner during your stay.

Whether you pack enough clothes for your entire stay or not is up to you. There are self-service laundry facilities at each resort, as well as a washer and dryer inside the one- and two-bedroom deluxe villas.

Shoes are another item to consider. It is wise to bring at least two pairs of tennis shoes for exploring the parks. With all the walking that occurs in the parks, blisters can happen. Being able to switch shoes allows your toes and feet the reprieve they need. Bringing a pair or two of sandals would be a plus for going to the pool or a short walk around the resort. (It is not recommended you wear your sandals all day in the parks unless you are used to wearing them during a long walking session.) Depending on your dining schedule, a nicer pair of shoes may be needed as well.

More must-have items include your toiletries. The basics include shampoo, body soap, toothpaste, toothbrush, lotion, makeup, and hair products. Items beyond those listed above depend on each person. Resort toiletries are provided and vary according to resort category. Value resorts typically provide soap, lotion, and a shampoo/conditioner combo. Deluxe resorts provide more toiletries.

When it comes to touring the parks, there are a few items to consider. Sunscreen is a must! The last thing you want is to be uncomfortable due to a sunburn. Another great item is a small backpack (or similar bag) to carry some essentials through the park such as granola bars, water bottles, sunscreen, camera, etc.

Disney welcomes you to bring food in the parks. Feel free to pack some of your favorite snacks so that you can eat them on the go. Another great option is Garden Grocer **gardengrocer.com**. This Orlando-based service allows you to choose grocery items online that you can then have delivered to your room. Since each resort now has a mini-refrigerator, you can have refrigerated items delivered to your room for your stay. Bell Services will hold your items until you arrive. They will even keep your cold items cold or frozen for you.

In this age of technology, bringing your electronics is a must. Your cell phone, laptop, tablet, camera, and iPod are items that you may choose to bring along. There is a small in-room safe for items you may not have with you at all times. Don't forget to bring chargers. Having a camera that only lasts for one day will not be fun. Also, bring extra memory cards for your camera because there will be a lot of photo opportunities.

This is just the beginning when it comes to packing for vacation, so there are a few packing lists in the appendix or sign up for the Magical Miles email list (**http://bit.ly/MagicalMilesList**) to get a printable version.

Packing for the Race

You may be a pro at packing for vacation, but packing for a destination race can be difficult. There are many items to consider, especially for a longer race.

If you are flying, it is highly recommended that you have all of your race essentials in your carry-on luggage. Lost luggage occurs, so make sure running items you cannot replace are with you at all times. If you are driving, you may want to keep your race essentials in a separate bag or suitcase for easy access.

Shoes. Don't forget your running shoes. You have trained long and hard in those shoes and forgetting them could throw you off your game. If you are running multiple races, it is advised you bring at least two pairs of shoes. The last thing you want is to run in wet shoes from rain during the first race.

Outfit/Running Clothes. There may be a favorite shirt that you want to wear for your race. Or maybe you even created a fun costume to run in. Be sure to bring a t-shirt/tank top, sports bra, shorts/skirt, and socks for race day. Also, make sure you complete one or two test runs in any new clothes you bought specifically for race day. You will want to be aware of any discomfort, chafing, etc., that may occur. Be sure to bring clothes for any type of weather as you never know what will happen on race day. Runners participating in cold weather races may be tempted to over-dress for race day. In order to prevent over-heating, you should be slightly uncomfortable (i.e., too cold) just before the starting gun goes off. Walkers may want to dress on the warmer side.

Hat/Visor/Sunglasses/Poncho. If it is sunny or rainy, making sure your eyes are protected will make your run more comfortable. Pack a hat or visor even if you don't think you may need one. If you aren't sure if you will need it the whole race, bring one you can toss if needed. It will be picked up along the course and given to a local charity. If rain, sleet, or heavy wind is predicted, then a poncho or a trash bag will provide some protection from the weather while you are in the corral. In the case of cold weather, duct tape placed over the top vents of your running shoes can block wind and some rain until the weather warms or subsides.

Running Gear. Runners are known for their gizmos and gadgets. Don't forget these on race day. If you have been training with a Garmin or other GPS item, be sure to bring it along. Another item is your iPod or mp3 player (for those needing music) along with your earphones. Be sure to keep the volume low so you can hear any course announcements. If your race is a longer distance, bring along some fuel. Be sure to bring what you have used during training. Popular items such as gels, sport beans or chews, and candy can be essential when you need a boost.

You may need something to carry your fuel in, whether it's a running belt or your hydration pack. In this pack, you can also include items you may need during the race such as blister packs, lip balm, Band-Aids, etc. If you have been training with a hydration belt, backpack or handheld, you may choose to bring it along for the race. This is especially important if you run with something besides water or Powerade.

Another must-have item is your ID. Sometimes things happen, and race officials may need to know who you are. You can bring your driver's license (a necessity for the after-party if you would like to buy an adult beverage) or wear your Road ID (or something similar). If you won't be meeting your friends or family after the race, don't forget your room key/MagicBand. If you plan on returning to your resort after a race through a theme park during park hours, don't forget your park ticket/MagicBand.

Camera/Phone. Disney races provide a lot of entertainment, and you will want to capture it. Bringing along a small camera or using the one on your phone is a great idea. Your phone also can let you communicate with your friends and family during and after the race.

Throwaway Clothes. Some Disney races occur in the early hours of the morning. This means that it may be a little on the cool side when you begin. Bring along a sweatshirt and sweatpants that you can wear to the corral and then toss to the side before the race starts. The volunteers will pick up all of the tossed clothes and donate them to local charities.

Bag Check. Prior to the race, you have the ability to check a bag. This allows you to bring items that you may need before or after the race, but not during the race. The bag is given to you at the expo along with your bib number to attach to the bag. This is the *only* bag you can bring to bag check, so don't forget it on race day.

Items to bring in your bag include a sweatshirt for after the race (especially for the cooler months), face wipes, your room key, phone, sandals or another set of socks and shoes, and even a fresh set of clothes. If there is a food that sits well with you after a race, it may be wise to put it in the bag as well. This bag is large, so feel free to fill it as much as you need. If you have any gel ice packs or other items that may be deemed concerning inside your bag, make sure to let the bag check attendants know prior to checking your bags. All checked bags are subject to canine search, so leave the any questionable items and pet treats at home.

If you are participating in a post-race party, you may want to put a backpack inside your checked race bag. You will not be allowed to return your bag to the bag check area once you've claimed your bag. The clear drawstring race bags provided by runDisney are spacious but also difficult to carry while touring a park for a post-race party. Place a drawstring backpack inside your checked race bag and use it to carry your items after you claim your bag. You may also use the locker rental in the parks, but lockers are subject to availability and cost between $7 and $9 with a $5 key deposit.

There is also a race day packing list in the appendix for you to use or sign up for the Magical Miles email list (**http://bit.ly/MagicalMilesList**) to get a printable version.

Krista & Megan's Tips

- Pack your race clothes, gear, and shoes in your carry-on. These are the items that you absolutely need for race day, so make sure they get to Disney with you!

- Prepare for all weather conditions. Florida weather can be finicky, so bring clothes for warm, cold, rainy, humid, or sunny.

- If you are participating in a runDisney challenge or multiple races, pack double/triple/quadruple of everything. It doesn't hurt to bring a little extra as well! Also be sure to pack recovery items such as compression gear, Epsom salts and a foam roller.

- Remember – nothing new on race day! Stick to the fuel, clothing, hydration system that you have been using during your training.

- Start creating a stash of throwaway clothes to use to keep warm before the race. You can also visit a local Goodwill to pick up items. We have seen sweatpants and sweatshirts, snuggies, blankets and even doctor scrubs! All clothes thrown to the side will be donated to local Orlando charities.

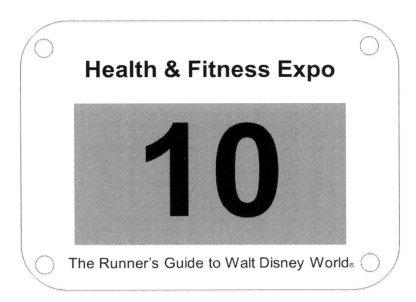

Health & Fitness Expo

10

The Runner's Guide to Walt Disney World®

The official start to a runDisney event weekend is the Health and Fitness Expo.

The Health and Fitness Expo occurs for all runDisney events. The expo is located at Disney's Wide World of Sports. What's important about the Health and Fitness Expo? Race bibs and shopping!

If you are a new to running then you might be wondering if attending the expo is necessary. The answer is yes! You must make plans to attend the expo to pick up your race packet, per the updated rules beginning in 2015.

Expo Preparation

Prior to event weekend, you will receive periodic emails from runDisney including Final Race Instructions and the Weekend Program. Runners should not underestimate the importance of the Final Race Instructions! Be sure to read through the information in its entirety. Specifics related to course changes, event transportation, and up-to-date instructions are included in this valuable document. Being very familiar with the Final Race

Instructions information prior to the events of the weekend will help your runDisney experience go smoothly. A virtual goody bag is also included in your email. Be sure to check the bag often as it is updated with special offers as your event gets closer. These offers continue up to a month following your event.

Prior to arriving at the expo, all runners and ChEAR Squad participants will need to print their waiver. Waivers are downloadable from the runDisney website approximately one month prior to race weekend. By entering your name and birthdate, you will be able to print your waiver, which includes the race you signed up for, your name, shirt size, and, most important, your bib number. Bib numbers indicate which corral you will start in on race day. If you want to find out what corral you are in prior to picking up your bib, you can use your bib number on your waiver and cross-reference with the corral placement lists located on the runDisney website. (Note: Corral placements are only available for the longer distances, specifically the half-marathon, marathon and challenges.) Looking up your corral prior to the race start is not necessary because your corral letter will be printed on your bib.

You will also want to look over the Weekend Program prior to your arrival. The program is available on the runDisney website and includes information about the race weekend and a map for the expo. This is important as you can see what vendors will be available. If you are at all strapped for time, make a note of what vendors you definitely want to check out. The program also includes a schedule of the speakers for the expo and maps of the Family Reunion area for the race.

Getting to the Expo

For those staying at a host resort, motor coach transportation is provided to the expo at the front of your resort. You can also choose to drive your own vehicle to the expo. Follow the signs to the ESPN Wide World of Sports Complex. Wear comfortable shoes to the expo because parking and bus stops are quite a long walk to and from the expo.

Packet Pickup

The expo starts at the HP Field House where you get your race bib and any commemorative items you may have purchased. There are booths split up by race event and your bib number, which appears on the waiver you print out prior to arrival. (If you don't have your waiver, no worries. There are computers and printers available for you to use. Do keep in mind that the lines for these computers may be long during peak times.) At the booth, you will be asked for your waiver and ID. You then receive your race bib and commemorative items. Your race bib will have a letter on it placing you in a corral for the start of the race. Starting in 2015, you MUST pick up your own race bib. A parent or guardian will be required to pick up bibs for children who are participating in the Kids Races.

A new policy is now enforced for those participating in any challenge, including the Coast-to-Coast Challenge. After receiving your race bib(s), you also need to get your photo taken. Look for the signs directing you to the location of the photo area. Once you completed your race, they will check your photo and race results prior to giving your challenge medal. At the expo, be sure to ask if you need your photo taken if you are participating in any type of challenge.

If you signed up for Race Retreat or signed up your family for the ChEAR Squad or Kids' Races, those items will need to be picked up as well. Head to the booths for those events, and don't forget your waiver and a photo ID. If you signed up for multiple races such as the 5K and half-marathon, you will need a waiver for each race. All runDisney challenges, such as the Dopey Challenge, Goofy's Race-and-a-Half Challenge, Glass Slipper Challenge, and the Dark Side Challenge only require one waiver.

For the larger events, your race shirt may be located in the HP Field House as well. When you pick up your race bib, they will advise you on where to pick it up.

There also may be official runDisney race merchandise inside the HP Field House. You can check out the availability, however the bulk of the official merchandise is inside the Jostens Center. If you purchase at the HP Field House and find something you like better in the Jostens Center, you do have the option to return your item, no matter which location it was purchased at.

> I just loved the Health & Fitness Expo. I really enjoyed all the support and encouragement from all the people selling their items. The area they could use more work on is to have more official race merchandise as it sells out quickly. The tip I would give is to get to the expo as early as possible.
>
> *Patricia, NY*

Vendors and Speakers

After you have your race bib, Race Retreat, ChEAR Squad, Kids' Races and any other pre- or post-race items, you can head into the main event at the Jostens Center. You will walk into the building on the second floor, looking down at the many vendors. Each expo is slightly different when it comes to vendors, but you can be sure there will be many of your favorite apparel and shoe companies, official race merchandisers, food sellers, and much more. Talk with the vendors, and maybe you will walk away with a new pair of shoes, new running clothes, yummy food, and much more. Many vendors offer great deals for the expo only, so if there is something you have been eyeing, now will be your chance! Just remember not to try out anything new on race day. Save your new purchases for later.

The most popular booth at the expo will be the runDisney official race merchandise. When it comes to the runDisney merchandise, it goes extremely fast. If you are looking for a specific shirt, Dooney & Bourke bag, or sticker for your race, it helps to go to the expo right away. Runners interested in having the best shot at purchasing race commemorative apparel should make travel plans to arrive on the first day of the Health and Fitness Expo. Many items sell out on the first day, and by the last day of the expo only a few commemorative items in odd sizes will remain. It is recommended you head straight to the main merchandise area first, located in the Jostens Center for most race weekends.

Another option is to have a friend or family member get to the expo early for you to grab must-have runDisney merchandise. They can bring in their phone to snap photos of the items to send to you or call you in regards to colors, etc. All runDisney apparel is currently Champion brand, so size accordingly. Unisex (or men's) sizing is true to size for men and runs large for women. Women's sizing tends to run small.

Certain race merchandise can be pre-ordered. In the past, this has included commemorative pins, necklaces, ear hats, Dooney & Bourke bags and even jackets. If you want to ensure you get any of these items, be sure to pre-order. It is worth mentioning that the design of most of these commemorative items is not known until you pick them up.

The Dooney & Bourke bags always sell fast, as well as any anniversary year commemorative items. In 2013, New Balance unveiled runDisney shoes, which have sold out at each expo in a matter of hours. At past expos, the number of shoes was limited to two pair per customer. It appears that new models will be released each year, so come prepared. In 2014, New Balance tried out a virtual queue in which you signed up, then were notified when it was your turn to go to the New Balance booth. Be sure to read your Weekend Program and keep an eye on **runDisney.com** for more information before any expo.

Also, be sure to go to the far end of the expo floor to pick up your race shirt and bag check bag. If you feel the size of your shirt may be incorrect, try it on right away. There is a shirt exchange table where you can trade your shirt for another size if that size is available. Since it is an exchange, keep trying back throughout expo hours as the size you want may suddenly appear. Shirt exchange may only occur during the latter part of the expo. Double-check when you pick up your shirt for the exchange times.

There are also various speakers and panelists throughout the expo that give forty-five-minute seminars. These seminars focus on training, racing, and nutrition. A popular speaker is Jeff Galloway, the official training consultant for runDisney. Past speakers have included runDisney nutritionist Tara Gidus, Ali Vincent from *The Biggest Loser*, Dimity McDowell and Sarah Bowen Shea from the book *Run Like a Mother*, along with former Olympians and elite runners. If you have the time to listen, these speakers will give invaluable advice! Another favorite is race director Jon Hughes and his team, who often give hints and tips regarding the course.

The schedule of the speakers is included in the weekend program that you receive via email prior to the event (as well as on **runDisney.com**). You will want to look this over prior to going to the expo as there may be a seminar or two you won't want to miss.

For those wanting to cheer on their runner, be sure to head to the Inspiration Station. This area includes poster board and markers for you to create a fun sign to support your runner and the many other runners along the course.

Once you have walked through the expo completely, it is time to head back outside and catch the bus to your resort. For most races, the expo lasts for multiple days, so feel free to head back again, especially as the expo can be quite crowded.

> I studied the list of companies who be present, I visited their websites and then marked what booths I wanted to make sure I visited. I did set a budget as well to keep me on track.
>
> *Sandi, AK*

Krista & Megan's Tips

- Arrive early. Arrive early. Arrive early. Yes, there will be crowds early on, but if you want *any* runDisney merchandise, you need to arrive early to get it! Another tip: head to the runDisney merchandise area in the Jostens Center *before* getting your bib.

- If you would like to experience the expo with smaller crowds, mid-afternoon may be best. This way you can visit the vendors without being shoulder-to-shoulder.

- To enjoy the expo to the fullest, leave the kids with a family member or friend. No strollers are allowed inside, and trying to keep the kids together (or entertained) while you look at running gear may prove to be quite difficult.

- It is anticipated that New Balance will release new shoes each year. If you are interested in purchasing a pair, be sure to sign up in the virtual queue.

- Do you have an Annual Pass? In the past, a small discount has been offered to Annual Passholders in the runDisney merchandise booth. You can also use Disney Gift Cards there as well.

- If you are running a little short on time, be sure to read the Official Race Program prior to going to the expo. Inside will be a map showing the vendors and the speaker schedule. This way you can plan out what areas you want to hit!

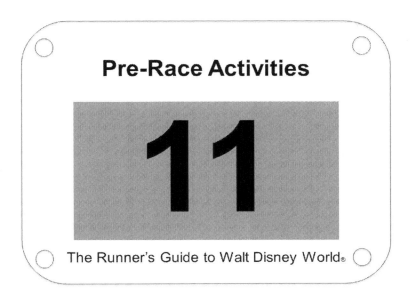

Pre-Race Activities

11

The Runner's Guide to Walt Disney World®

For those wanting a fun way to enjoy the Disney magic during a runDisney event, there are pre-race activities available for select events. From pre-race meals to Race Retreat, these separate ticket events offer an exciting way to start your race weekend.

Pasta in the Park

Pasta in the Park is a pre-race meal option available for the Walt Disney World Marathon Weekend and the Princess Half-Marathon Weekend. It is a separate ticketed event costing $54 per adult and $30 per child aged three to nine. (Children under three years of age are free.) Tickets must be purchased in advance as they tend to sell out prior to the event.

This event begins at 7 p.m. in Epcot on the night prior to the race. (For the Walt Disney World Marathon, it occurs on three evenings, Thursday, Friday, and Saturday. For the Princess Half-Marathon, it occurs on Friday and Saturday evenings.) The dinner is held in the Wonders of Life Pavilion located near the United Kingdom pavilion and includes various types of salads, pasta, and dessert served buffet-style. A live DJ will keep the energy high as your favorite Disney characters put in their appearance. Kids' activities include

Hula Hoops and dancing near the stage. After dinner, you can watch Illuminations: Reflections of Earth from a private reserved viewing location at World Showcase. Keep in mind that Illuminations does not start until 9 p.m., so it may be 10 p.m. or later by the time you get back to your resort.

Trying to decide if Pasta in the Park is an event you want to attend? Think about your race the next morning. It will be an early wake-up call, and this event is later in the evening, especially if you stay for Illuminations. Also, the food is a standard pasta buffet. You may be better off eating an earlier dinner on your own.

Pre-Race Taste

Wine & Dine Half-Marathon Weekend includes a Pre-Race Taste event the night prior to the half-marathon. Tickets are $79 for those three and older. (Children under three years of age are free.) This private event takes place from 6:30 p.m. – 8:30 p.m.

Located in the Indiana Jones Epic Stunt Spectacular Theater in Disney's Hollywood Studios, this private party includes early entrance to the park, tastes from the Epcot International Food and Wine Festival, a drink coupon, cash bar, and appearances from your favorite Disney characters.

One nice aspect is that the half-marathon isn't until the following evening, so the time of the Pre-Race Taste isn't an issue as it is for Pasta in the Park.

Race Retreat

Race Retreat is a fun extra for participants and Platinum ChEAR Squad members for race mornings. Costs for runners start at $120 and go up to $230. Race Retreat is only available for the Walt Disney World Half-Marathon, Walt Disney World Marathon, Goofy's Race-and-a-Half Challenge, Dopey Challenge and Princess Half-Marathon.

Pre-Race

Before the race (starting at 3 a.m.), runners participating in the Race Retreat can wait inside the temperature-controlled tent while enjoying a pre-race meal of bagels, fruit, coffee, water, and Powerade. There is also a padded stretching area that allows you to prepare for your race, along with a private bag check. However, the most important feature is the private port-a-potties. There is no need to stand in a long line for the port-a-potty prior to the race start. While the port-a-potties are of the same type provided outside Race Retreat, the lines will be significantly shorter inside Race Retreat, and they are usually well stocked with paper products. Hand washing stations are also available.

Post-Race

After the race, participants are treated to a hot brunch (including cocktails for those interested) with unlimited water, soda, and Powerade. Should you wish to change out of your race clothes, a separate changing tent is available. You can also check your official results via the computer terminals hooked up to the Internet to allow runners immediate access to race results.

Feeling the post-race aches and pains? There is an area to self-treat any injuries you may be experiencing, or you can pay just $10 for a ten-minute professional massage. Keep in mind the massages usually require you to sign up, so be sure to do so prior to your race to ensure you get one.

Need a little entertainment after your race? Various characters participate in the Race Retreat fun! Get a photo with your new medal around your neck. You can also watch a live feed of the finish line. Watching the participants smile, high-five, hug, and even cry as they cross the finish line is amazing to see.

Participants of the Race Retreat also are given a commemorative item such as a towel, socks or flip-flops.

Trying to decide if Race Retreat is something you want to do? Think about the uncertainty of the weather. This is the primary reason for choosing Race Retreat, especially for the winter month races. If the Race Retreat is still available, expect it to sell out immediately if the ten-day forecast calls for bad weather.

If you have family members or friends, they can join you in Race Retreat after your race (or while you are running) if they purchase the Platinum ChEAR Squad package. More information is available in Chapter 17.

Race Retreat is becoming more popular and selling out quicker, especially with the new challenges. The percentages only appear on the registration page for the event, so be sure to keep an eye out to ensure they don't fill up before you've registered.

> Race Retreat was awesome. To have somewhere to sit down and get ready where there were lights and not mill around in the dark was great. I liked the quick bag check before and after the race as well. After the race, we hung out at the race retreat and had breakfast. It was great to get out of the sun and watch people finish on the live feed on TV. I also had a massage. Later, I used the changing tent to clean up and we went straight to Epcot for a few hours.
>
> *Jeanne, DE*

Krista & Megan's Tips

- While these events can be fun with a group, they are by no means necessary. They do offer easy access and unique experiences if your family is interested.

- Keep in mind that the Pasta in the Park Parties are offered later in the evening. If you plan on eating and staying for Illuminations, you may not get back to your room until after 10 p.m. This is not ideal with a 2:30 a.m. wake-up call the next day!

- If you have dietary restrictions, be sure to let someone know upon your arrival for any of the meals or Race Retreat. A chef will prepare food that is safe for you to eat.

- Race Retreat is wonderful for the Walt Disney World Marathon in particular! Having a place to (try to) relax before the race is nice, but, more important, having a place to cool down after the race is fantastic!

- If you would like your family or spectators to join you in Race Retreat after your race, be sure to get Platinum ChEAR Squad for them. This way they can eat and celebrate with you!

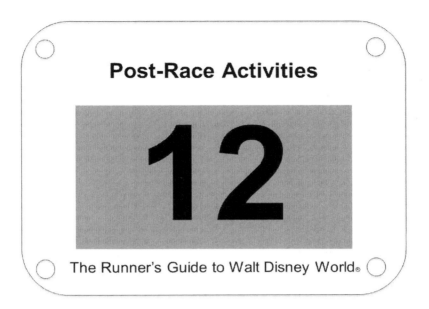

Post-Race Activities

12

The Runner's Guide to Walt Disney World®

You've trained hard. You've put in the mileage. You finished the race. Now it's time to celebrate! A few races offer after parties and events that are open to all participate.

Post-Race Breakfast

After the 5K and 10K races during Marathon Weekend and Princess Half-Marathon Weekend, you can enjoy a post-race breakfast. This is a separate ticketed event costing $40 for adults and $30 for children, ages three to nine. (Children under three years of age are free.)

> We loved the breakfast! The morning was very cold and it was perfect to be able to get some breakfast, meet some characters and reunite with our non-runner family members.
>
> *Kami, TN*

At a post-race breakfast in the Family Reunion Area (most recently, inside the Race Retreat tent), your family can enjoy a buffet along with Disney character meet-and-greets. Included in the breakfast buffet are fruit salad, quiche, breakfast burritos, french toast sticks, sausage links, pastries, juice, and coffee. This is a great way to get breakfast directly after your race, but some runners may choose to go back to their resort, shower, and head to a special breakfast in the parks or at their resort instead.

Post-Race Parties

Disney Springs Cool-Down Party (WDW Marathon Weekend)

For the Walt Disney World Marathon Weekend, enjoy a fun after party in Disney Springs on Sunday evening starting at 2 p.m. Enjoy food and music while you unwind after your big race. This event is open to runners, their families, and the public at no charge. Special offers are also given at select locations by showing your finisher's medal.

Happily Ever After Party (Princess Half-Marathon Weekend)

Similar to the Cool-Down Party during Marathon Weekend, the Happily Ever After Party will be held in Disney Springs on Sunday evening. Starting at 2 p.m., runners, their families, and the public can enjoy food and music as racers show off their new medals. This event is free for all.

Finish Line Party (Wine & Dine Half-Marathon)

Want to experience the International Food and Wine Festival in a fun way? Then the Finish Line Party after the Wine & Dine Half-Marathon may be just for you. Participants in the half-marathon get access to this party with their race registration. Friends and family wishing to join can purchase a ticket to this event. Admission starts at $75 per person. Ages three and under are free. Tickets will sell out as the event approaches. Make sure you purchase tickets, especially if you have spectators that are interested in attending the event following the race.

The Finish Line Party allows early access into Epcot at 7 p.m., where you can watch the runners start and finish with live viewing locations. (If you wish to watch your runner cross the finish line, head to the Epcot parking lot. As long as you have your ticket, or race bib for runners, you will be able to enter the party afterward.)

Attractions are also operating during the Finish Line Party, and with little or no wait you can enjoy Soarin, Test Track, and Mission: Space. You also have access to over twenty-five Food and Wine Festival Marketplaces, as well as a $15 gift card to use at vendors located throughout the World Showcase. There is a festive environment at this after-party, which includes live music performances, a DJ, and much more. Don't forget the appearances from your favorite Disney characters. This party goes until 4 a.m., so you can celebrate your race until the early morning hours!

We love this party! It is the highlight of the entire weekend to me. I have seen characters every year, and love to ride Soarin and Spaceship Earth with my medal on. The food is exceptional after the race, but this year the weather just about robbed me of the fun since I was chilled and my feet couldn't get dry. I'll definitely consider doing it again.

Dara, SC

Krista & Megan's Tips

- This is a fantastic way to celebrate your accomplishment! All Wine & Dine Half-Marathon participants will gain access to their respective after parties with their race bib.

- If you have spectators, family members, or friends who didn't participate (or participated in Mickey's Jingle Jungle 5K), they will need to purchase a party ticket. Watch the capacity levels as the parties can fill up quickly!

- For a few of these after parties, the race course goes through the park. There are cast members that re-direct the race course so you can pass through. However, we found that it can take up to 20 minutes for the re-direct to occur, so be prepared!

- Be sure to pack an extra set of clothes, including a jacket or sweatshirt for the after parties. After your race, it can get a little chilly while enjoying the park.

- Don't forget your medal when attending the parties at Disney Springs. Discounts may be available for runners who show their medal!

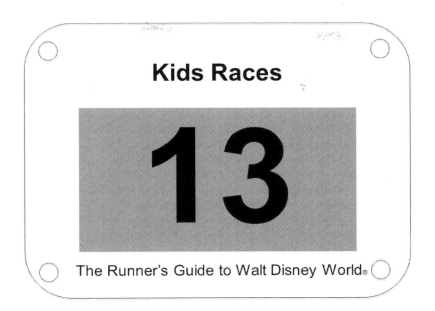

Kids Races

13

The Runner's Guide to Walt Disney World®

Disney Kids' Races provide even the smallest tike an opportunity to participate in a race. From the Diaper Dash (twelve months and under) to the Mickey Mile (thirteen and under), all kids can have fun running a race of their own.

While the runDisney 5K runs have been deemed a family event, there was a change in 2015. Participants must be at least five years of age on race day and able to complete the event on their own. If your child will be too young, or if 3.1 miles is a little daunting, the Kids' Races are highly recommended.

> My grandson loved his race and hi-foured mickey! He loves doing them.
>
> *Lisa, TX*

Getting to the Races

Those participating in the Kids' Races should arrive at ESPN Wide World of Sports (or Epcot in the case of Princess Half-Marathon Weekend) no later than one hour prior to the posted start time of the

Kids' Races. These races happen quickly, and all kids should be in their assigned corral no later than fifteen minutes prior to the race start. One parent should accompany small children in the corral and may run with their child during the race. Keep in mind, there may be a wait involved before the races start. This can be uncomfortable if weather is poor.

Pre-race activities include music and tents with coloring sheets and other kid-friendly activities. Since Kids' Races occur in stages, these activities are essential in keeping the kids entertained while they wait.

It doesn't matter which race weekend you are attending; all Kids' Races offer the same events. However, in the past, Kids' Races may be executed differently depending upon how they are staged in the pre-race area. In the past, Kids' Races that are run on the track at ESPN Wide World of Sports (such as during Marathon Weekend and Wine & Dine Weekend) are better organized and more efficiently executed. However, there have lengthy wait times that can prove difficult for little runners.

Mickey Mile

The Mickey Mile is a one-mile run for children thirteen and under. The Mickey Mile is a timed event where all competitors are winners, so no awards are given out. Finisher medallions will be given to all children who participate. Parents may run with children but will not receive a medal. Participants can view their official race time at **runDisney.com**.

During Princess Half-Marathon Weekend, the Mickey Mile race course includes a section inside Epcot. This is a great opportunity for kids to experience the excitement of running inside a park.

Dash Events

Kids' Dashes are held for babies through children aged eight. The following age groups participate in the distances listed below:

100m Dash: 1-3 years old
200m Dash: 4-6 years old
400m Dash: 7-8 years old
Diaper Dash: 12 months and under

Each age group has a corresponding start line. Look for the flag color that corresponds with the number or color on your child's race bib. These events are not timed, and official race results are not recorded. Parents are encouraged to run with their children. Please make sure your child is wearing their official race bib prior to the race start. There will be a tear tag that parents will use to claim their children from security if you choose not to run with your child. Children will not be allowed outside the secure race area without an adult with a matching tag. Volunteers will be on hand to direct parents and children prior to and immediately following the races. The Diaper Dash takes place at the finish line immediately before or at the conclusion of the Kids' Races.

After the Race

As your little one crosses the finish, make sure they give Mickey (or another Disney character) a high-five. Official race photographers are located throughout the Mickey Mile and the Dash Races to photograph your little one in action. Parents can also get a great shot along the course or at the finish.

If you did not run with your child, you will need to claim your child using the tear tag from your child's bib.

Krista & Megan's Tips

- Kids' Races are a great bargain! For the cost of entry, your child will receive a race-themed character t-shirt. The price of race entry is worth the t-shirt alone!

- There is a cap on each dash. While the registration page may show availability for Kids' Races, the dash for your child's age group may be full. Sign up early to guarantee availability. These races do tend to sell out close to race weekend.

- Costumes are welcome! You'll see many kids dressed in their favorite costume, so don't hesitate to pick a costume that goes with your racer's running shoes.

- If you are headed to the expo on a day the Kids' Races are going on, be sure to stop by and cheer the little runners on!

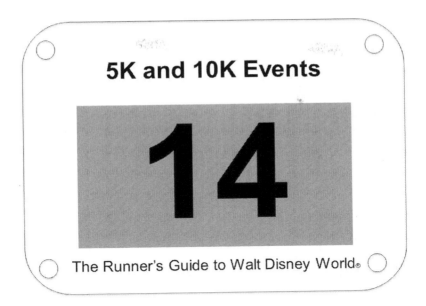

5K and 10K Events

14

The Runner's Guide to Walt Disney World®

A 5K or 10K race is a great way to dip your feet into the running game or experience a runDisney even with the whole family. Below you will find information to calm any concerns so you can enjoy your moment with confidence.

Course Information

Family Fun Run 5K (January) and Royal Family 5K (February)

These 5Ks follow the same route, starting and ending in Epcot. The race begins in the parking lot area for the first stretch of the race. The course enters World Showcase in between Mexico and Norway near Mile 1. You then continue clockwise through World Showcase and through the International Gateway at Mile 2. The course continues backstage for a short distance and then comes back into World Showcase near Canada. You continue toward Future World, past Spaceship Earth, and around the park entrance. The course exits near Universe of Energy at Mile 3, and then it's the home stretch to the finish line.

Walt Disney World 10K (January) and Enchanted 10K (February)

These 10K races held in Walt Disney World also follow the same course. They begin in the Epcot parking lot area, at the same start as the 5K. The course veers left (as opposed to right during the 5K) and heads onto the nearby highways for the first two miles. There is a sharp hairpin turn just after the one mile marker, followed by a hill (overpass) before heading back to Epcot.

Just after the 3 mile mark, the course enters World Showcase in between Mexico and Norway. You continue clockwise around World Showcase, exiting at the International Gateway. The course then makes a left as you run around the Boardwalk area (be careful as the wooden boardwalk can be slippery), around Crescent Lake and past the Yacht and Beach Club.

The course continues back toward the International Gateway, going backstage. You return into Epcot near the Land, cut through Future World and past Spaceship Earth. It is a quick jaunt backstage before heading to the finish line.

Star Wars 5K – The Dark Side (April)

New in 2016 is the Star Wars 5K in Walt Disney World. At the time of publication, the only course information is that the race begins and ends in Epcot. Be sure to check **runnersguidetowdw.com/course-maps/** for up-to-date information about the course.

Star Wars 10K – The Dark Side (April)

New in 2016 is the Star Wars 10K in Walt Disney World. At the time of publication, the only course information is that the race begins in Epcot and ends in ESPN Wide World of Sports Complex. Be sure to check **runnersguidetowdw.com/course-maps/** for up-to-date information about the course.

Mickey's Jingle Jungle 5K (November)

Experience Animal Kingdom before the park opens during this 5K race. Start in the Animal Kingdom parking lot and head toward the park entrance and past the Tree of Life. The course then takes you through Africa and on toward Asia, past Expedition Everest. You then will run through DinoLand USA and back into the parking lot for the finish.

> It was amazing! I ran the 5k in the morning and the half that night. I was completely exhausted but all the cheering cast members and volunteers kept me moving forward
> *Aimee, MI*

Pre-Race Information

The 5K races are great for families, new runners, veteran runners, or those wanting to get in as much Disney mileage as they can throughout the weekend. The 5K races at Walt Disney World provide an entirely different experience from the longer distances. Beginning in 2015, 5K participants must be at least 5 years old on race day and able to complete the race on their own.

The 10K races were new in 2014. These races provide a great bridge between the 5K and half-marathon distances. As with the 5K events, the experience is one you will never forget.

Night Before the Race

All 5K and 10K events occur in the morning. Therefore, make sure you prepare the night before. Lay out your clothes, fill out the back of your bib with your emergency information, and set multiple alarms. This will ensure you aren't scrambling early in the morning. If you are checking a bag, place your sticker on your race bag the night before.

Getting to the Race

If you are staying at a host resort, arriving at the race is easy. Bus transportation begins two hours prior to the event. Although you do not need to be at the start line as early as for the distance events, it is best to arrive at least an hour in advance. Whether you are driving, taking a cab, or using race transportation, be sure to allow yourself enough buffer time. There will be plenty to do when you arrive. Coffee stations and picture opportunities are located throughout the pre-race area. Lively entertainment will keep you going until it's time to head to your corral. If you are checking a bag, allow plenty of time to find the bag check area. Only the clear plastic bag provided at the race expo may be used at bag check. Make sure you attach the sticker, which matches your bib number, to your race bag. Do not include any valuables in your checked race bag.

Bathrooms

Bathrooms in the form of port-o-potties will be located throughout the pre-race staging area and on the course. Keep in mind the lines will most likely be quite long, so get in line right away.

Corral Placement

Your bib will indicate your corral placement for the 5K. In the past, start line corral placement is based upon your expected finish time, and you will be placed into a corresponding pace group. However, lately there has been no rhyme or reason in terms of 5K corral placement.

For the 10K events, you will enter an estimated pace at registration. From this pace, you will be assigned a corral. The corral is indicated on your race bib with a letter. Be sure to go into the correct corral for the safety of all participants.

For both the 5K and 10K races, there are approximately five corrals. They are released every eight (or so) minutes. Keep in mind that although an estimated pace was given at registration, these corrals aren't very accurate.

> This was my first 5K ever. I couldn't believe how organized everything was. From the buses to the hotels to the race, it was fantastic!
>
> *Laurie, GA*

The Race

Ready. Set. Go!

It's race time, and 5K races are considered fun runs. Race results are not posted and awards (other than a participant's medallion) will not be given out, so relax and enjoy your run.

The 10K races are timed, though many still run these races for fun. Awards and race results are given for the 10K race. Headphones are discouraged for both race distances due to audio messages throughout the race course.

For the runDisney challenge events that include the 5K or 10K races, a large portion of the race field will include those challengers. This is something to keep in mind if you are a first-timer or if you are running with children.

Bathrooms

For the 5K events, port-o-potties are available at the start and finish area. There are also real bathrooms available inside the parks.

The 10K events also will have port-o-potties available at the start and finish areas. Since the race course includes Epcot, there are real bathrooms available along the course. The race course also includes the Epcot resort areas, so you are able to run into the resort lobby for a pit stop if needed, but this will take you off the race course path.

Water Stops

During the 5K races, there will be two water stops. These stations will only include water. If you have been training with a drink other than water, you will want to bring your own hydration. Since all 5K race courses include a park, you can also stop at water fountains if needed.

For the 10K race events, there are three water stops. These stations only include water, so plan accordingly, especially if race day is warm or humid. If you have been training with your own hydration pack, you may want to use it to ensure you have water or electrolyte drinks available whenever you may need them.

Characters

Characters are typically found throughout the 5K and 10K events, so don't forget your camera. From time to time special characters will make an appearance, especially if there is a theme to the race. Be sure to take advantage of these great photo opportunities. The lines for the characters may get long, but they usually move fairly quickly.

Photographers

Official race photographers are also located throughout the course and at the finish line. Make sure your bib number can easily be seen so that you can locate your pictures after race weekend is over. At any character location, most photographers (or the runner behind you) will take a photo with your camera as well. Have your camera ready to go and limit it to one photo to keep the line moving quickly.

Safety

Throughout the race, medical personnel on bikes will ride along the course. Alert personnel if you need medical assistance. A medical tent is also located at the finish line. Runners should be able to maintain a sixteen-minute-mile pace (or faster if you would like to include stops like character photos). Anyone who is unable to maintain this pace may be picked up and transported to the finish line area. Effective 2014, there is no longer a stroller division within the 5K races.

Finish

The finish line is in view. Cross it with a smile on your face!

After the Race

You've done it! Cross the finish line and claim your medal! All 5K participants will receive a finisher's medallion made of a thick rubber material and 10K participants will receive a finisher's medal (similar to the distance race medals) at the completion of the race. After you cross the finish line, you will receive a snack pack with packaged snacks and fruit. Powerade and bottled water is also provided. Check out the locations for photo opportunities with your medal throughout the race area. Live entertainment continues for at least an hour post-race. Make sure you pick up your bag from bag check by 9 a.m., or you will need to find Lost and Found to claim your bag. Once you are ready to go back to your resort, head to the parking lot for post-race transportation. Buses to host resorts will be located near the Family Reunion Area. Cabs are also available.

A post-race breakfast is available after the January and February 5K and 10K races. Tickets must be purchased in advance. (See Chapter 12 for more information.)

Krista & Megan's Tips

- Remember, the 5K is not a timed event. Although you can time yourself, you will not have a time associated with your race bib.

- The 5K race includes a medallion, but it is not made of metal as for the other races. The 5K medallion is made of a rubbery material, but still has a great runDisney design to it!

- The 10K race also includes a medal that is similar to those earned during the half-marathon and marathon events. The medals always take the design of the race theme and in the past, have been unveiled by runDisney a few months before the event.

- During the January 5K race, a large percentage of the runners are part of the Dopey Challenge. Be sure to keep any children close by to avoid trampling.

- Prepare for long character lines, especially during the 5K events. The lines usually move fairly quickly, however there will be waiting involved.

- For these shorter distances (especially the 5K), many runners are running for fun and do not have a time goal. If you are looking to run a personal record during the 10K, do you best to get to the front of the corral as there can be some course crowding.

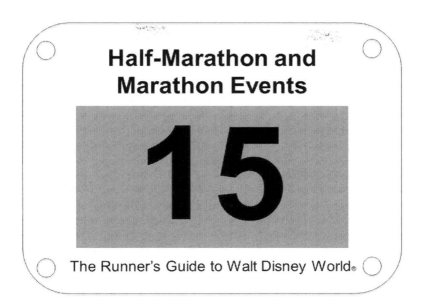

Half-Marathon and Marathon Events

15

The Runner's Guide to Walt Disney World®

You clicked register. You trained for months. And now the time has arrived.

Course Information

Wondering where your race will take you? Here is a look at each race course and special items to note.

Walt Disney World Half-Marathon and Princess Half-Marathon

These races follow the same course. The race begins along Epcot Center Drive for the first 1.5 miles. From there you will make a sharp right-hand turn onto World Drive. Keep in mind that it will be dark during this portion of the race. Watch your footing carefully, especially along the lane markers on the road where there are raised bumps that you can easily trip on. Also be aware when you enter the Magic Kingdom gates as there are large speed bumps.

While on World Drive, you will run through the Ticket and Transportation Center. This is not only full of great spectators, it is also a great chance to use real bathrooms. After exiting the Ticket and Transportation Center, you will head toward the first hill under the Seven Seas Lagoon. Be sure to look up at the great DJ giving you the extra push you need. After conquering the hill, you will run by the Contemporary Resort and toward a backstage area of Magic Kingdom. This area can cause congestion, so be prepared to slow down a bit.

You will enter the park near Town Square and make a sharp right onto Main Street USA. The crowd will be loud as you get your first glimpse of Cinderella Castle! Smile as you run along Main Street USA and make a right toward Tomorrowland. This is another place to stop at a real bathroom. From Tomorrowland you will enter Fantasyland and listen as the trumpeters welcome you to Cinderella Castle. Run through the castle, staying to the left for a great photo opportunity, then head into Liberty Square and Frontierland. This is your last chance to make a pit stop at real bathrooms for a while. Pass by Splash Mountain and into another backstage area.

From here you will run on the service road behind the Grand Floridian Resort & Spa. Watch your footing as the path narrows. After passing by the Grand Floridian and Polynesian Resorts, it's back onto World Drive for almost three miles. A fuel station with gels will be available for those needing an extra boost. Note that the water station is around a half mile after the gel station.

Around Mile 10 comes one of the toughest parts of the course, the banked onramp. The camber of the road is quite steep, so stay to the right to save your leg muscles. As you run across the overpass, be sure to look to your left to see the crowd of runners below. There are two more overpasses to conquer (without cambered roads), and soon you will see Epcot.

Run through a parking lot area and enter Future World in Epcot. There are real bathrooms, so take advantage if needed. Next you will run toward World Showcase, turning around before the lagoon. Run back through Future World, taking a right into another backstage area. In this area is a fantastic entertainment area, giving you the boost you need for the last section of the race. A few quick strides and you will see the finish line! Smile big as you cross the finish line and accomplish your goal.

> I loved how organized the start was and the finish. Nicely done, Disney, nicely done!
>
> *Laurie, GA*

Walt Disney World Marathon

A new race course was unveiled in 2013. The course initially follows the same route as the Walt Disney World Half-Marathon and Princess Half-Marathon through the service road behind the Polynesian Resort.

After leading you past the Grand Floridian and Polynesian resorts, the race course takes you to the Walt Disney World Speedway. There is a hill getting into the speedway, so be sure to watch your step, especially if there is dew on the ground that morning. You will run along the track with a few special guests to keep you entertained.

Upon exiting the speedway, you will run along service roads toward Animal Kingdom. Along these roads is a fuel station that includes bananas and gels. The road does pass by the sewage treatment plant, so prepare your nose for a smell.

The course will enter Animal Kingdom near Rafiki's Planet Watch and then through Asia. This is another chance for a real bathroom stop. The course takes you by Expedition Everest, and if the park is open, you can take a quick ride! Run through DinoLand USA, and then out to the parking lot area, crossing the halfway point of the race, and past the park entrance.

Next up is Osceola Parkway. The road includes a few overpasses, but it's important to note that there is virtually no shade from this point of the course through to the end. After a two-mile run along the Parkway, you will enter ESPN Wide World of Sports Complex. This is another opportunity to take advantage of real bathrooms. This three-mile stretch winds around various sports fields and tracks and through Champion Stadium, home of the Atlanta Braves' spring training. The complex includes narrow paths and uneven ground at times, so be sure to watch your step. There is also a fuel station that includes bananas and gels for those needing a pick-me-up.

Once you exit the complex, you will begin your trek to Hollywood Studios. There is a hill in the form of an onramp as you head past the park sign. You will enter the park behind Tower of Terror and continue backstage for a while. The course enters the park in the Streets of America, where you will get a sugar rush to help you through the last few miles. Take advantage of real bathrooms if needed. There is a tunnel area (past where they create costumes) and you may lose signal on your GPS. You will run along Hollywood Boulevard and through the entrance of the park.

Next is the path along the water toward the Boardwalk area. After passing by the Boardwalk, you will see a small hill toward the Yacht and Beach Club Resort. Run along the resorts and toward the International Gateway into Epcot.

Upon entering Epcot, you will make a right, run through the United Kingdom, and continue counterclockwise through the countries of World Showcase. This is another chance to use real bathrooms if needed. After running through Mexico, you will make a right toward Future World. Exit the park to the right, take in the fantastic entertainment, make a few small jogs, and see the finish line. Smile as you cross the finish line!

A few items to items to consider are the Walt Disney World Speedway and Hollywood Studios. The Speedway has been closed, which may impact this race course. Also, Hollywood Studios is undergoing a major refurbishment with the additions of Star Wars Land and Toy Story Land, which may impact the course as well. Stay tuned for more information.

Star Wars Half-Marathon – The Dark Side

New in 2016 is the Star Wars Half-Marathon event in Walt Disney World. At the time of publication, the only course information is that the race begins in Epcot and ends in ESPN Wide World of Sports Complex. Be sure to check **runnersguidetowdw.com/course-maps/** for up-to-date information about the course.

Wine & Dine Half-Marathon

The race begins at ESPN Wide World of Sports Complex. Run along Victory Way, then make a left onto Osceola Parkway. This road includes a few hills in the form of overpasses. Follow the road for another two miles, and then watch the speed bumps at the Animal Kingdom entrance.

Run through the parking lot area and enter the park. Be careful as the paths inside the park are uneven due to the park's theme and can be a little tough on the legs. Take advantage of the real bathrooms if needed. The course takes you past the Tree of Life, through Africa, toward Asia, past Expedition Everest, and through DinoLand USA. From there you will exit the park and run through the parking lot area.

It's back onto Osceola Parkway for another two miles. Make a left onto World Drive, heading up an onramp toward Disney's Hollywood Studios. Along the road is a fuel station with gel for those needing it. You will enter the park near the Tower of Terror, running along Sunset Boulevard and on through Pixar Place. If you need a pit stop, take advantage of the real restrooms. Enter backstage areas, then run on through the Streets of America where the Osborne Family Spectacle of Dancing Lights will be lit up! Run behind the Indiana Jones Stunt Spectacular and through the park entrance. From here you will run along the path toward the Boardwalk area. There is a slight hill as you head toward the Yacht and Beach Club areas along Crescent Lake. Enter Epcot through the International Gateway, heading backstage. You will come into the park near the Imagination Pavilion, running by The Land. Run through Future

World, taking advantage of real bathrooms if needed. Continue backstage, make a few strides, and the finish line will be in view. Make a sharp left and cross the finish line with a smile!

One item to note is that Hollywood Studios is undergoing a major refurbishment with the additions of Star Wars Land and Toy Story Land. Also, in 2015, the Osborne Family Spectacle of Dancing Lights will be making their final debut. It is expected to impact the race course, so stay tuned for updates.

> I especially loved the people staying at the Epcot area resorts who set up with signs along the course to cheer. Many didn't even have a racer in the race, but were there to encourage total strangers! It actually made me emotional when a woman I didn't know shouted that she was proud of me! Definitely magical!
>
> *Holly, NY*

Runner Etiquette

During a race, there are thousands of other runners with you. It is important that you follow proper race etiquette in order for everyone not only to be safe, but also to experience a truly magical race. The biggest piece of advice is to be aware of yourself and the runners around you. Below are great rules of thumb for all runners to follow.

- Pay attention to pre-race instructions. This will help guide you during the race and keep you safe.
- Run or walk no more than two across.
- If you are walking in a group, please start in the last corral.
- If you are stopping at a water station, move all the way over to the table. Grab your water and move away from the table, leaving a path open for others to get water as well.
- Stay to the right unless you are passing others. Also stay to the right during a walk break.
- If you are going to be taking a walk break, raise your hand to indicate you are coming to a stop or slowing down.

- Try not to come to a complete stop along the course, or do so on the side of the course. Let those behind you know that you will be stopping.
- If you need to get around someone, feel free to give a little, "Excuse me," or, "Coming through." If someone behind you says this, move over to the right to let them through.
- Watch your elbows. Areas of the course can be narrow, and you don't want to jab someone.
- If you need to get rid of an item, make sure to throw it completely off the course so that others don't step or trip on it.
- Say "Thank you!" to all the fantastic volunteers!
- At the end of the race, you may see your family members or friends. Keep in mind they cannot come onto the course. Give a little wave and smile and meet them after the race.
- When you have finished, keep moving forward. Don't stop in the finisher's chute unless it is absolutely necessary.
- Be courteous and don't take more water, Powerade, or snack boxes along the course or after the race than you need. It is recommended you only take one of each item, unless it is very hot or humid.
- If you are able, stay around to cheer on those who are still finishing!

No matter what, the key is to create a magical experience for yourself and the other runners. The Golden Rule "Do unto others as you would have others do unto you" always applies!

Pre-Race Information

Night Before the Race

Believe it or not, the race actually begins the night before. By making sure you are ready the night prior, you not only have peace of mind, but you may be able to sleep in longer and enjoy the parks a bit more.

The first thing you should be doing the day prior is hydrating. Keep that water bottle close by and refill it often. If the weather is particularly hot and humid, it would be wise to add in electrolyte drinks for extra hydration.

Next is to lay out your race clothes. Make sure you include everything, from shoes to sunglasses, underwear to watch, fuel to race bib. Have it all in one location where you can just grab it and put it on. This is a great time to double-check that you haven't forgotten anything.

Be sure to fill out the back of your race bib. Although we don't want to think about it, sometimes unfortunate incidents occur such as an injury or illness. The back of the race bib will allow medical personnel to know your history and contact your family.

Now is a great time to attach your (filled out) bib to your clothing. Safety pins will be in the clear bag you receive at the Expo. Make sure it is visible for the race. (And don't worry if it's not straight. That is a tough art to master.) Try not to bend or break the strip along the back of the bib as that is the device that will time your run.

And finally, it is time to set the alarms. Yes, those morning races require an early wake-up call. It is wise to set multiple alarms, along with a wake-up call from the front desk. You sure don't want to sleep through the race. Be sure to allow yourself plenty of time to get up, get ready, and get to your mode of transportation to the race. If you decide to take a nap before an evening race, the same suggestion applies.

Getting to the Main Event

It's race day! After months of preparation, the most important thing now is getting to the race on time. Disney races have a fantastic start, complete with entertainment and fireworks for each corral. This is one thing you don't want to miss. Yes, those morning races are early. But finishing your morning race early allows for a post-race nap and leaves you with plenty of time to visit the parks. So, set your alarm (or two) and get ready to race. Runners should plan to arrive at the race location at least 1.5 hours prior to the race start. It is recommended you get to the bus stop early as lines can become quite long. If you are driving, always allow more than enough time as road closures and traffic backups do occur.

Once you arrive, you should check your bag and begin the walk to your corral. There will be a security check prior to the Family Reunion area. Anyone with a bag of any kind (including hydration belts, etc.) will be required to go through this checkpoint.

For morning races that start at Epcot, you will be walking approximately fifteen to twenty minutes to the start. This walk can be congested, so please, *please* err on the side of caution and give yourself plenty of time to get to the race start. If you anticipate needing a pre-race restroom break, give yourself some extra time as the lines for the bathrooms will be long. Runners need to be in their corrals by at least a half hour prior to the race start, or you will not be allowed to start.

For the Wine & Dine Half-Marathon evening race, runners need to be in their corrals by 9:15 p.m. for a 10 p.m. start. However, the last bus leaves the host resorts at 8 p.m. Always allow extra time and get to the staging area and corrals early. The walk to the corrals is much shorter for these races and there is a large, grassy area for you to sit and relax before the race.

Due to increased security, you cannot walk to the race from your resort. Failure to abide by this rule can result in disqualification from the race as you will not be able to start. You must enter through the staging area, then walk to the corrals from there.

Pre-Race Activities

Wondering what you will do for an hour or two before the race? No worries. Disney will keep you entertained. At the Family Reunion (or staging) area, a DJ will be playing music to get the adrenaline pumping. Take this time to check your bag, do some light stretching and, of course, use the restroom. Don't fret, the entertainment will continue once you get to your corral. This is also an opportune time to eat your pre-race snack.

Bag Check

You may want to bring some items you will need after the race but don't want to carry while you're running. These items must be placed in the large clear bag you received at the expo and held until the end of the race. In the staging area, find the letter of your last name and give your bag to the volunteers. When you are finished with the race, you can head back to the bag check area to pick up your bag. Keep in mind that bags may be searched or inspected for your safety.

Not sure of what to include in your bag? Just look at the packing section and appendix for some ideas. As a reminder, you can only use the clear bag you received at the expo for bag check and must affix the sticker that matches your bib number. Don't leave anything valuable inside the bag check bag.

For the Wine & Dine Half-Marathon, just drop off your bag at the start, and it will magically be transported to the finish area for you to pick up.

Bathrooms

Port-o-potties will be located throughout the pre-race area for both runners and their family members. Runners who have purchased admission to the Race Retreat will have access to private restrooms. There are also port-o-potties just beyond the bag check area.

Please note, that there will also be port-o-potties located at the start (as well as en route to the start) so do not delay in heading to your corral as there are usually plenty of bathrooms. The line for port-o-potties in the pre-race area often causes significant congestion for runners walking to the corral area, so be prepared.

Port-o-potties will also be located throughout the race course. And, although no one may admit it, there are times when a runner "heads to the woods" before, as well as just after, the race starts. Yes, the area near Epcot is heavily wooded. Use your discretion, but it's a fairly common occurrence. It is worth repeating, it is wise to tuck some extra tissues in your pocket or running belt.

Getting to the Start

Once you arrive at the race (whether by car or race shuttle) for the morning races, there is a bit involved with getting to your actual corral. Again, allowing plenty of time to get to your corral is extremely important. For most Disney races, you will be required to walk to the starting area, which takes an average of fifteen to twenty minutes. The walk may be congested with other runners, so be sure to allow yourself enough time.

For the evening races, the walk to the corrals is much shorter. Be sure to use the restrooms before getting into the corrals.

Corral Placement

Anyone searching on a message board regarding Disney races will soon realize corral placement is one of the most highly discussed issues of Disney races. After registering for your race, a link will become available on runDisney.com (under the race weekend you are participating in) where you will input your proof of time. To enter this proof of time, you need to have completed a race of a specific length in order to qualify for a possible lower corral placement. You must give a valid proof of time or you will be placed in the last corral. It is important to be honest as corrals are also for runner safety. (See Chapter 4 for more information on updating your proof of time.)

Each race has a wave start where runners are split into multiple corrals. The beginning corrals have a smaller number in each corral, increasing through the last corral, which is the largest. The corrals are released one at a time with roughly three minutes between the earlier corrals, increasing to six or more minutes between the later corrals. For the safety of all participants, it is necessary that you stay in the corral marked on your bib. Participants are allowed to move to a corral with a slower pace without being officially reassigned; however, runners should never attempt to move forward.

There are several hundred runners in each corral, and there will be numerous corrals for each race. Your race bib will have a letter indicating your corral placement. Corrals are indicated by giant signs at the race start. Your race bib will be checked by a cast member before you are allowed entry into any corral. If you are wearing layers prior to the race start, make sure you can show your bib with minimal effort. Remember, your race bib should go on the layer you expect to wear for the majority of the race and not on any "throw-away" clothes that you wear pre-race.

Elite runners will be in the very first corral. These runners are seeded and in competition to win the race. This group will be followed by Corral A, Corral B, and so on. Usually, Corrals A and B contain runners who have a fast race qualifying time. All corrals will be seeded with the exception of the last corral, which will be for those who do not submit a qualifying race time.

Runners and walkers with higher expected finish times will be placed into higher corrals. Don't stress if this is your first race and you are placed into a higher corral. Many participants become overly concerned with their corral placement and its relationship to finish time. Your timing chip will start as soon as you cross the start line, which will give you an accurate race time. There's no need to worry about the sixteen-minute-per-mile time limit and your corral placement. Even if you are the last person across the start line, as long as you have trained for a fifteen-minute-mile or faster, you will be fine and may even have some time to take a couple pictures with the characters and stop for a bathroom break. (Keep in mind that lines may be long, so if you are interested in many photo stops, train for a faster pace.)

Once you've found your corral, settle in and enjoy the entertainment. A few of your favorite characters may even come and wish you luck. Fireworks send off each corral in grand style. There are numerous Disney characters, the national anthem, inspiring stories televised on a Jumbotron, and, before you know it, you will be on your way.

I enjoyed it when the DJ led the last two corrals in Don't Stop Believing as we prepared to start. It gave me a boost! I took the trip with my daughters and everything was near perfect.

Patrice, IL

The Race

This is it, the moment you have been training for. With the bang of the fireworks, you are off.

Congestion

Depending upon the race you are running and your corral placement, it is highly likely that the first mile or two will be very congested as everyone tries to find their pace. The runners will start to spread out as the race goes on. As a general rule, the slower runners should stay to the right so that it is easy to pass on the left.

There are areas where the course narrows, which usually results in tight quarters. Stay calm and try to keep your pace. Know that the course will widen back out, giving everyone more room. During some races, such as the morning half-marathons, runners will experience congestion at different race points due to course narrowing throughout the entire race.

If you are walking with a group or using a run/walk combo method, it is recommended that you stay to the right. Walkers and runners should not span more than two people wide to allow space for faster participants to pass on the left.

For those using the run/walk method, it is also recommended you raise your hand prior to beginning a walk interval. This indicates to those behind you that you will be slowing down.

Another thing to consider is that it may be dark during your race. There are lights along the course (as well as some large and very bright spotlights), but you still need to be careful. Try to stay on the road so that you are aware of your footing. Note that there are lane markers that stick up from the road. Be careful. Watch for course announcements warning of narrowing or bumps.

Removing Layers

For the morning races, it is quite possible that it will warm up as you run along the course. Feel free to remove extra layers, but be sure your bib is always on the outside. Discard your layers along the side of the course, and volunteers will pick them up and donate them to local charities. Always be aware of those around you as you discard.

Characters

Yes, there are many characters along the course. There are can be over twenty photo opportunities for the half-marathons alone. (And that's just the characters. Don't forget about park landmarks.) From the classic princesses to villains, at least one of your favorites will be along the course.

Past characters include Mrs. Incredible, Princess Tiana, Lilo and Stitch, Captain Jack Sparrow (complete with his pirate ship), Mushu, Chip 'n Dale, Darkwing Duck, the Mad Hatter, and many others.

And don't forget about the end of the race. A few special characters may be waiting just for you at the finish line.

Although the lines for the characters may look long, they tend to move quickly. If you are worried about your time, choose the characters you want to see most.

Bathrooms

Don't worry; there are bathrooms available along the course. Port-o-potties are strategically located near the water stations, so be sure to look at the course map to stay aware of their location.

There are even real bathrooms available inside the parks. See the above Course Information for hints as to where these are located. However, we are all runners and do know that sometimes nature calls at inconvenient times. No one will judge if you need to run off the road into the woods!

Photographers

You may bring your own camera or phone for some great photos along the course. And there are also official photographers along the course as well.

If you are familiar with Walt Disney World, then you have probably experienced PhotoPass photographers in the parks who take your picture with characters or in front of Disney landmarks. PhotoPass photographers will scan a PhotoPass card or your MagicBand to save your pictures and allow you to purchase them at a later date. It is important to note that PhotoPass photographers are **not** the photographers you will encounter on the race course. For more information on PhotoPass photographers, see Chapter 19.

Photographers from MarathonFOTO will be all along the course snapping pictures of you while running or with characters. You can even stop at park landmarks for some great photos as well. Be sure to smile when you see a photographer. You *are* in the Happiest Place on Earth.

A few tips:

- Photographers are usually located along popular spots. Think Cinderella Castle, the Epcot entrance, etc. Look out for them and prepare in advance for your pose. Check the MarathonFOTO website or their booth at the expo prior to your race as they may include a map with photographer locations.
- There may be a MarathonFOTO photographer with each character, but they will take a photo with your camera as well if you ask. (The runner behind you may take it for you as well.) If race pictures are important and you want to save money, bring your own camera. Do keep in mind that it may be dark outside during your race, which will affect the quality of your photos.
- If your course goes through Cinderella Castle, upon exiting, go to the left to get a great photo in front of the castle.
- Make sure your bib number is clearly showing. This is the way you will be identified in your photos. The last thing you want to do is sift through the thousands of unidentified photos to find yours.
- Be prepared: the photos are expensive. You can look at pricing prior to your race at **MarathonFOTO.com**
- A photo and possibly video are taken as you cross the finish line, so smile big. You can also get a finisher's photo taken after receiving your medal, which is a great keepsake.

Water, Powerade, and Gels

Water stations are located approximately every 1.5 miles along the course. Take advantage of them. Powerade (usually lemon-lime) will also be at the stations, so be sure to listen to what liquid you are being handed. If they are offering water at the first part of the stop, Powerade will usually be at the second half of the stop and vice versa. If you have been training with a hydration belt or pack, you may still want to bring it along. This ensures that you have liquid whenever you need it and will not need to wait for a station. Be courteous to the runners behind you and don't take more than your fill.

For the longer races, Clif gels are offered. Located around Mile 9 for the half-marathons, you can grab your favorite flavor to get the fuel you need to get you to the finish line. (If you have been training with other fuel, bring it along with you.) The marathon offers multiple fuel stations to help push you through 26.2 miles, including bananas, gels, and even chocolate.

Medical tents are also available at various locations along the course. If something doesn't feel right, stop and talk to a medic. These stations also have Vaseline (for the areas that are rubbing together too much), aspirin, and Biofreeze (for the achy areas).

> I thought the water stops were really well placed and I took advantage of them all. Thankfully I read that gels weren't being handed out until mile eight so I carried my own fuel with me to take at mile six since I needed the fuel earlier than mile eight.
>
> *Emily, MO*

Mile Markers

Even the mile markers along the course have Disney magic. Each marker includes a scene from your favorite Disney movies. This is another great photo opportunity. Cast members and/or official photographers are typically not found at mile markers. However, you can usually find another race participant who has stopped for a photo and is willing to help you out.

On each mile marker will be a timer. Keep in mind that this is the time from *when the first corral started.* Your personal time does not start until you cross the start line. A good tip is to look at your watch/phone when the first corral starts, then look at it again when you cross the start line. This will give you a good indication of how many minutes to subtract from the mile marker timers so that you can keep a better idea of your overall time.

Spectators

Throughout your race, there will be many spectators cheering you along. Located throughout the parks and areas near resorts, friends and family members of fellow runners will come out to encourage you during your race. Other spectators include cast members and even some local residents who have come out just to give you a smile.

And don't be surprised if you hear your name called. If you register at least a month prior to the event, your name will be printed on your race bib, allowing spectators to cheer for you by shouting your name.

> All the people who came out to cheer, I applaud you!!!
> *Pamela, IL*

Volunteers

Whether it is helping you into your corral, handing you water, or putting a medal around your neck, there are various volunteers throughout your race experience. These volunteers are giving their time to make your race even more magical. Be sure to give them a high-five or tell them thank you. They truly can give you the extra push you need.

Injury or Illness

What happens if you get injured or feel ill while on the course? No worries, Disney will make sure that you are safe.

Along all the courses are multiple medical tents. If something does not feel right, please stop and talk to one of the medics. They can assess your situation and help you determine how to proceed.

If you are not near a medical station, there are still volunteers, Disney cast members, and other runners available to assist you. (The running community is amazing. Many will stop to ensure you are okay.) Along the course are cyclists that carry medical supplies, including an automated external defibrillator. Flag down one of these cyclists, and they can assess the situation.

If there is an emergency of any kind (to yourself or another runner) and medical help is not nearby, please call 911. Your call will be not only get immediate attention, it will also be called into the team supporting the runDisney event. There are multiple ambulances along the course, so help is never far away.

It cannot be stressed too much: if you feel that you are injured or sick, please stop along the course. You do not want to make it worse. A medical staff member will come to you to assess the situation and determine the next step. Past runDisney events have endured high heat and humidity, so be sure to listen to your body.

Time Limits/Sweeping

There is a time limit for the course as you will be running along roads throughout the Walt Disney World Resort. This time limit is approximately 3.5 hours for any half-marathon and seven hours for the Walt Disney World Marathon. The time limit starts when the last person crosses the start line. If you have been training for a fifteen-minute-per-mile pace, you should not be worried.

In the back of the pack are two pacers with balloons, also known as the sweepers. There are also two cyclists with orange flags. As long as you are in front of these volunteers, you will be fine. These pacers start after the last person crosses the start line and keep a sixteen-minute-per-mile pace throughout the course. They will not only let you know if you are in danger of being swept, but they will also offer you encouragement along the way.

Keep in mind, there are no safe points along the course. The time limit applies until the finish line. For example, even if you are two miles from the finish line, if you do not keep the sixteen-minute-mile pace, you can still be swept. There are no guarantees extra time can be given to you as Disney needs to clean up the roadways and course.

If you fall behind a sweeper, a bus will be available to take you back to the Family Reunion area. Do not be discouraged. A Did Not Finish is always better than a Did Not Start. You can always sign up for another race.

> Once again, I found the race weekend to be busy, but streamlined. Great on-course support, there were plenty of amenities for us slower runners and the energy was fantastic!
>
> *Heather, NH*

The Big Finish

The moment has come. You can see the finish line. And you cross it. Smile big. Cry a tear. And then celebrate.

After you cross the finish line, volunteers will put that amazing runDisney medal around your neck. Wear it with pride. From there you can have your finisher's photo taken: a moment to cherish forever. If you participated in a runDisney Challenge or are receiving your Coast-to-Coast medal, be sure to get in the appropriate lines to get those medals. A volunteer will check the photo you took at the expo, ensure it is in fact you and hand you your medal. If you completed the first leg of your runDisney challenge, go to the appropriate line and follow instructions so you can receive your medal upon the completion of the challenge.

Next are the tents. There are multiple tents, so be sure to check them all out. One will have food, including a box with goodies that include allergy-free items. (The contents of these boxes changes with each race, so if you are used to a certain food after a run, pack it in your bag check bag.) You can also grab some water and Powerade. Next are the medical tents. Medics are available to assess any problems you are feeling. There are also self-help areas where you can get ice or Biofreeze. The important thing is to keep moving, unless you are truly not feeling well or are hurting a lot.

Beyond these tents is the bag check area. Using your bib number, the volunteers will get your bag.

For those who have the Race Retreat package, you can go back to that tent for some pampering. Enjoy a light meal, get a massage, and even change out of your race clothes.

For those wanting another great keepsake, you can get your medal engraved. In the Family Reunion area is a location where you can get your name, date, and finish time engraved on your medal. Cost is around $20, so be sure to tuck some cash in your running belt or bag check bag.

There also may be a merchandise tent in the Family Reunion area. It includes leftover merchandise from the Health & Fitness Expo, related to the race weekend. It never hurts to take a look inside, although the contents are usually very picked over.

After the Race

Once you have received your medal and food, you will head to the Family Reunion area where you can meet up with your family and friends. There are large signs with letters, so be sure before the race to agree on a letter at which to meet up.

If you participated in a morning event, you will most likely want to either head back to the resort for a shower or find some food. If you stayed at a host resort, bus transportation is available back to your resort. (More information is provided in Chapter 8.)

If you participated in an evening event, it is time to party. For the Wine & Dine Half-Marathon, you will end in the Epcot parking area, where you can then head inside Epcot for the Finish Line Party. Medical tents are located in this area for those needing them. Changing tents are also available after you claim your bag in the Family Reunion area. Keep in mind, once you exit the finishers chute area, you cannot re-enter. You can then head into the park to ride the attractions and enjoy the Food & Wine Festival booths.

> Live in the moment and cherish each moment. It is meant to be fun so let it be and don't stress the small stuff.
> *Casey, FL*

Krista & Megan's Tips

- Listen to the announcements in the family reunion area before the race. They will let you know when it is the last chance to drop off your bag at bag check, what corrals need to head to the starting area and other important information. And, yes, the port-o-potty line is long, but get in it even if you don't have to go!

- Bring your own fuel! Even if you have trained with the same product runDisney is offering (usually Clif gels), you may need fuel earlier in the race. Tuck some extra fuel in your pocket or running belt just in case.

- RunDisney events are not usually conducive to personal records. Although they are possible (many have done it), with the characters, narrow areas, and large amount of runners, it is best to consider these events fun races. Get that PR on another course that isn't as entertaining!

- Train for at least a fifteen-minute-mile pace (if not faster). This will ensure you have time to stop for character photos, take a potty break, and still be ahead of the pace requirement.

- Be prepared for any kind of weather. Past races have included sleet, heavy rain, high humidity, etc. Adjust your goals based on weather conditions.

- Keep a positive attitude! Not only will it make your race more magical, but also all of those around you.

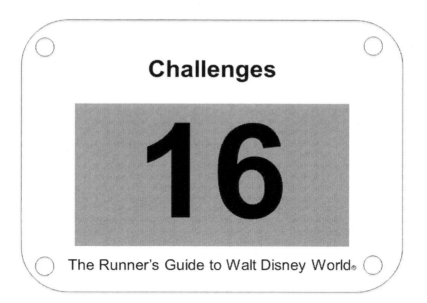

Challenges

16

The Runner's Guide to Walt Disney World®

It all started with Goofy's Race-and-a-Half Challenge, where participants complete the Walt Disney World Half-Marathon on Saturday followed by the Walt Disney World Marathon on Sunday.

The past couple of years, runDisney has continued to add even more challenges to their schedule. With the addition of the Dopey Challenge, Glass Slipper Challenge and Dark Side Challenge, runners are upping their game. These back-to-back races include a lot of preparation and dedication both before, during, and after the events.

Training

Completing one 10K, half-marathon, or marathon can be daunting enough. Completing two within twenty-four hours of each other (or four within seventy-two hours) is a whole new ballgame. Thankfully, there are a few training plans to help ensure your body is prepared before the big race weekend.

RunDisney Training Consultant Jeff Galloway creates training plans for all runDisney events. He also has created training plans for the challenges, adding in back-to-back runs throughout the training cycle. All challenge plans are aimed at finishing in the upright position, focusing on training smart and avoiding injury. His recommendation is that participants walk the first day and run or run/walk the second day. (Keep in mind that the more experienced runners may be able to run/walk or run both days. Listen to your body to determine the best method for you.) These back-to-back runs are key to your challenge training. A challenge is not the time to slack off on your training plan.

These challenges are intended for runners with previous distance race experience, so be sure to take a look at your past training to ensure you will be able to handle the training and races before signing up.

What to Pack

Since the challenges include two (or four) races, you need to make sure you pack accordingly. Use our packing lists found in Chapter 9 and the Appendix, and double (or quadruple) items for the challenge you have selected.

It is also recommended that you bring two pairs of shoes. Sometimes blisters or uncomfortable areas can appear during a run, so having another pair to wear during your second race is a good idea. Make sure you have broken in both pairs of shoes prior to the event. Some running experts recommend breaking in two pairs of the exact same model of shoe, which ensures your running form remains the same.

Along with multiple running outfits, be sure to bring extra fuel. Within the challenge, the distances double on the subsequent day, so it is wise to bring more fuel than you think you will need.

As with any race, prepare for all weather conditions. With the challenges, it may be sunny one race and rainy the other. Or it may be cold both races. Bring enough gear for any type of weather during all events.

Since you will need to recover properly between races, it is recommended you bring compression gear, Epsom salts, relief for blisters, sunburn or chafing, and recovery fuel. You may also want to bring a tennis ball or foam roller to roll out sore or tight muscles. The goal is to recover between races so you are ready to double your distance the next day.

As a reminder, you can always purchase items at the Health & Fitness Expo, but you don't want to try anything new on race day.

Before the Race

A few weeks after registration, you are able to submit a proof of time for corral placement. (See Chapter 4 for more information.) You also can send runDisney an updated proof of time before a specific deadline, usually a couple months before the event. This proof of time definitely helps as runDisney has been placing challenge runners a corral or two behind from normal. Since you may be starting slightly further back than normal, be prepared to deal with a little more crowding than you may be used to.

As with any runDisney event, it is wise to set out all of your gear the night before. Since the wake-up calls will be early during your challenge, you don't want to forget anything. Challenge runners will have one race bib to use for both races, so be sure not to misplace it. (For the Dopey Challenge, you will have two race bibs. One for the 5K and 10K, and another for the half-marathon and marathon. Make sure you know which bib is for which races.)

During the Races

While each race during your challenge includes its own fun entertainment and excitement, there are a few instances where the courses are quite similar. For example, during Goofy's Race and a Half Challenge, the first 8 miles of both races are identical. Prepare yourself in advance for a little bit of déjà vu.

If you have not participated in a challenge of back-to-back races before, it is wise to take the first race (or races) a little easier than normal. Always remember that the last race is the longest and you don't want to burn out your legs too quickly.

Remember that you are not alone! Each challenge includes thousands of other runners, enduring the same string of races. It is very common for you to look to your left or right and see a challenge race bib. This is a great way for you to make new friends, encouraging one another along the way.

Between Races

You have completed part of your runDisney challenge! Now it's time to rest those muscles in preparation for the next day.

Upon returning to your resort, you may want to grab some ice from the ice machine. If you have any areas that are bothering you, ice will calm down the inflammation. It is also recommended that you take an ice bath (or jump in the resort pool if it's cool) or a bath with Epsom salts.

To allow the muscles to recover, many runners utilize compression gear. Compression socks are highly recommended as they will help your calves, shins, and feet. Another option is compression shorts, which will help your thighs, quads, and gluteus muscles. Don't feel silly wearing them in the parks or around your resort. Everyone will see your medal and understand!

Although you may want to take a nap, it is actually better to walk around after the race. Head to a park for a couple hours, but take it easy. Enjoy your surroundings, go on rides that allow you to relax, and leave the park mid-afternoon at the latest.

After resting in your resort room, be sure to get dinner early. Load up on your favorite pre-race meal, then get to bed early. You will have another very early wake-up call.

It is common for the most difficult part of a challenge to be the consecutive early wake-up calls, especially for the Dopey Challenge. Do your best to get extra rest throughout the day.

> I did the Dopey Challenge and it was unlike any other race experience I have ever been a part of. The marathon was my seventh overall marathon, and even the three Chicago Marathons pale in comparison to the Disney Marathon.
>
> *Jeromy, IN*

After the Races

Congratulations! You are a runDisney challenge finisher! Enjoy your extra medal (or, in the case of the Dopey Challenge, medals) and wear them with pride.

Be sure to follow the same recovery steps outlined above. Your final race is the longest of all, so you want to make sure your muscles are well taken care of.

If you head to the parks, wear your medal! (It is recommended you only wear one, most likely the challenge medal itself. When multiple medals are worn around your neck, they clang together, which can cause the medals to get scratched. Not to mention, they are heavy!) This is a great opportunity to get character photos with your medal, a fantastic keepsake to bring home.

It's time to celebrate! Great ways to celebrate your accomplishment include:
- A post-race massage
- A celebration meal at your favorite restaurant
- A fireworks cruise

Krista & Megan's Tips

- The challenges do require a lot of training. Please keep this in mind prior to signing up. It is recommended that you have a strong running base prior to running these challenges.

- There are a very limited number of participants for each challenge. If the challenge is full, but the individual events are not, you can sign up for both events, but you will not get the challenge medal.

- Make sure that you train for back-to-back runs! By doing so, you know what you need to do between races to get your body ready for the next race (of double distance) the next morning.

- For the Glass Slipper Challenge, Dark Side Challenge and Goofy Challenge, you will use the same bib for both races. Do *not* throw it away! For the Dopey Challenge, you will use one bib for the 5K and 10K events and another for the half-marathon and marathon. Yes, it will be gross, but it allows runDisney to see that you have, in fact, completed all events for the extra medal.

- Packing for a challenge can be a little daunting. Use gallon-size Ziploc bags – one for each race. This way you make sure you have everything you need for each race, from clothes to fuel!

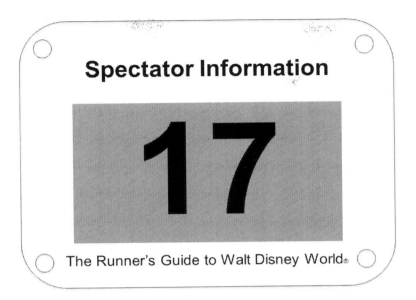

Spectator Information

The Runner's Guide to Walt Disney World®

While life is not a spectator sport, spectating can definitely be a sport when it comes to races at Walt Disney World! If you are attending a runDisney event, you may find spectating presents a logistical challenge. Supporting your runner at various points on the course is a fun and challenging way to enjoy a runDisney event. Here are several tips that can make cheering on your runner a more enjoyable experience.

Tracking Your Runner

Wondering where your runner is on the course? runDisney offers a service that will notify spectators via email or text message as their runner crosses specified thresholds throughout the race. Whether you are following a runner while at Walt Disney World or cheering them on from home, runner tracking is a great way to know where your runner is on the course. A few weeks prior to each runDisney weekend, runDisney will open registration on **runDisney.com** for this service that allows spectators and supporters to enter your cell phone number or email to receive live updates on your runner's progress at various points along the course. The best part about this is—it's *free*. Most races charge for this feature; however, runDisney wants to make this race as magical as possible and offers it to participants at no charge. Each text will include your time, pace, and estimated time of finish. The estimated time of finish is a definite plus for the spectators who want to be at the finish to greet their runner.

Another perk of runner tracking? If you want to let everyone know how you are doing in your race, you can even have your splits sent to your Facebook or Twitter account.

An example of the distance thresholds where runner notifications have been sent in past races are:
- 10K - 5K and Finish
- Half-marathon - 5K, 10K, 15K, and Finish
- Marathon - 5 miles, 10 miles, 13.1 miles, 20 miles, and Finish

At these thresholds, the text and email include time elapsed (since the runner crossed the start line), average pace, and estimated finish time. A great part about the estimated finish time is that it not only includes overall race time, but also the estimated time to expect the runner to cross the finish line! For example, a text may say a runner is expected to finish the race with an overall time of two hours and forty-five minutes and to expect them to cross the finish line (or ETA) around 8:30 a.m.

In past races, runner tracking at runDisney events has been fairly reliable. In some instances, text messaging is delayed due to poor cell reception or increased activity. These issues can result in receiving delayed messages. Therefore, it's a good idea to have a Plan B for tracking your runner, such as an app or communicating directly with your runner via text message or a phone call.

Additional tracking options include various apps on your smart phones. Apps such as Find My iPhone, Google Latitude, RoadID, and Map My Run have options where you can track your runner's phone. Keep in mind that some of these apps are not free. You will also need to be aware of the course map so that you know where your runner is based on road names and areas. It would be wise to test out these apps prior to your runDisney event, as they may not always be accurate or may drain the battery on the runner's phone. It is also worth noting that increased cell activity in race areas can cause interference with some of these apps.

> There were nine of us in our party and only three of us ran the half. I made sure to tell everyone where to go for the bus and where to meet us. They were able to find everything quickly and it was easy for them. Disney made sure to have clear signs with simple directions. There was enough space for them to see us and keeping track of us on their phones was very easy.
>
> *Christina, TX*

Encouraging the Runners

Whether waiting for your runner or just enjoying the race from a spectator perspective, you have the opportunity to encourage every runner that you see. Here are some ways to give the runners passing by an extra boost.

Support Signs

Creating a sign is not only a way to give your runner a boost they need, but will also encourage other runners along the course. All you need is a large piece of poster board and a marker. Come up with a fun saying or slogan, or even just a "Go Name Go." This will put a smile on your runner's face. You can even make a sign at the Inspiration Station at the Health and Fitness Expo.

Also know that *every* runner appreciates fun signs. Although you are there to encourage your runner, you may encourage others along the way. Incorporating pop culture or funny sayings into your sign will make the runners smile, just what they need when pushing through the pain.

Food and Candy

During the longer distances, runners need fuel to get them through the miles. A fun way to get the entire family involved is to bring candy to the course. You are sure to be popular when you hand out candy like licorice sticks and chocolate or salty snacks like pretzels.

One of the best places to hand out food and candy is around two to three miles from the finish. This is when runners can really use that last burst of energy to make it to the finish line.

Cheers and High-Fives

The runners pass by quickly, but hearing the cheers from the crowds is what keeps them going. A great way to interact with the runners is to cheer their name. RunDisney includes the runner's name on their race bib, which is an easy way for spectators to offer personalized cheers.

Another great way to get involved is to offer a high-five. It is sure to bring a smile to a runner's face when you are offering the encouragement they need to push through that portion of the race. (And it never hurts to have a cute kid be the one offering the high-fives!)

Spotting Your Runner

How do you spot your runner in a mass of over 20,000 other runners? And how does your runner spot you? You plan ahead! The night before the race, plan on a few locations along the course where you will spectate. This way, the runner will know where and on what side of the course you are so that they can look for you.

One of the best ways for your runner to spot you is to carry helium-filled balloons with you on race morning. Pick up at balloon at Magic Kingdom or Hollywood Studios (balloons are not sold at Epcot or Animal Kingdom) the day before the race. While helium-filled balloons are a tad expensive at Walt Disney World, one balloon will last through an entire week of races. A balloon will be the easiest way for your runner to spot you in a crowd of spectators.

Another option is to call or text each other at various mile markers or time frames. This way, beyond the runner tracking, you can get an idea of how far away they are from your location. Plan to call your runner or have them call you at specific mile markers before your planned meet-up locations. (Runners, be sure to move to the side and off of the road before texting or calling.)

Also know what your runner is wearing. This will help you pick out your runner in the midst of thousands of others. Bright colors help, but with the increase in colors of popular sports clothes, there may be many others in the same color top.

Based on their training runs, most runners know when and where they could use some support. Some runners will prefer to see their support team early in the course with a priority placed upon meeting up at the finish line. Other runners, such as marathoners, may prefer to have friends or family in the higher miles. In this case, it is extremely unlikely that you will make it to the finish line in time to see your runner finish.

If your priority is seeing your runner as many times as possible, for a half-marathon you should plan on one viewing location in the early/middle of the course, and then head to the finish line. For the full marathon, it is best to plan on two viewing locations in the first two-thirds of the race, and then head to the finish line.

Spectator Locations

Looking for the best locations to see your runner? Here are a few favorites by race event.

5K Races

Since the 5K races are usually within a park, the best location to see your runner is at the start and finish. (Spectators are usually not allowed inside the park for 5K events.) Or better yet, join your runner for this family-friendly event.

10K Races

Similar to the 5K races, most of the 10K race is also in a park. Since this race is longer, it not only goes through Epcot, but also around the Epcot resort area. Your family can watch the runners pass along the Boardwalk area or near the Yacht and Beach Club. You can also watch your runner from the start and finish line areas. Keep in mind there will most likely not be enough time to see them in the Epcot resort area as well as the start and finish. Note that only race participants are allowed inside the park during the 10K races.

Walt Disney World Half-Marathon and Princess Half-Marathon

These races offer the same course of a starting near Epcot, going through Magic Kingdom and back through Epcot. Great locations to spot your runner are at the Transportation and Ticket Center, in Magic Kingdom, near the Grand Floridian or Polynesian resorts, and at the finish line.

For those wanting to see their runner multiple times, we suggest choosing one of the following: Ticket and Transportation Center or Magic Kingdom Park or Grand Floridian/Polynesian resort. With any of these options, you should have enough time to make it back to Epcot for the finish. Spectators should plan on heading to their first viewing location by 5:30 am. If you are staying at a monorail resort, you can leave just prior to this time. If you are staying elsewhere, you will want to go to Epcot with your runner, and then get on the monorail from there.

Within Magic Kingdom, you can watch for your runner along Main Street USA with no park ticket required. Main Street is the only area available for spectators who are not a part of ChEAR Squad. This area can be quite congested, so you may need to adjust your location along Main Street accordingly.

For those participating in ChEAR Squad, you can see your runner before they head into Tomorrowland and when they exit Cinderella Castle. Note that the ChEAR Squad area will be very congested for spectators, and to have a good viewing spot, you should arrive at Magic Kingdom by 5 a.m. Magic Kingdom may not open until the race officially starts, but it is important to be in line before the park opens and then head directly to the roped-off ChEAR Squad area to stake out your spot. One of the advantages of arriving so early is that you will be able to see the race leaders as they run through the castle. This is great entertainment while waiting for your runner to arrive.

At the Transportation and Ticket Center, there is a long area for you to find a great spot to spectate. Find a spot along the fence and cheer loudly as runners come through!

Another location is behind the Grand Floridian and Polynesian resorts. Walk through the parking lots toward the back road and find a spot along the road. There is a roped-off area that you must stay behind. The road is narrow, so spotting your runner may be a little easier. (Tell them to stay to the left if possible.)

The finish line offers a great view of your runner as they complete their race. Keep in mind this area can become very crowded. ChEAR Squad has special seating and is usually less crowded than the general finish line seating grand stands. For spectators who are not a part of the ChEAR Squad, you can stand along the fences prior to the grandstands or sit in the stands behind the finish line. The stands behind the finish line are very crowded and offer no shade, which may not be ideal for kids.

Walt Disney World Marathon

The marathon offers more opportunities for you to spot your runner. The course starts the same way as the Walt Disney World Half-Marathon and Princess Half-Marathon, so see the above section for locations including the Ticket and Transportation Center, Magic Kingdom Park, and Grand Floridian or Polynesian resorts. Spectators could easily pick one of these spots and then head to the finish line or any spot in World Showcase.

Another great location for spotting your runner is at Disney's Animal Kingdom. The runners enter the park then come back through the parking lot, offering a chance for you to see your runner. Keep in mind that park transportation may not yet be available (depending on the speed of your runner), so driving your own vehicle or taking a cab may be necessary. This can be difficult or expensive due to traffic congestion and road closures, and is recommended for spectators staying at one of the Animal Kingdom resort properties. If your party has numerous spectators traveling, then Animal Kingdom is a great viewing location since it is typically the halfway point of the race.

The course takes the runners through the ESPN Wide World of Sports Complex. There are various locations to see your runner inside, including shaded areas so your family can stay comfortable. However, if seeing your runner finish is a priority, this location should be avoided. It is very time consuming to take the motor coach over to ESPN Wide World of Sports.

A fun place to watch the runners is near the end of the race. There is a lot of crowd support when the runners exit Disney's Hollywood Studios, along the path to the Boardwalk area and near the Yacht and Beach Club resorts. With only a couple miles left, this is where the spectators shine. Keep in mind that if you watch your runner here, you will not be able to make it to see them finish. This is also a great location for families with small children who are staying at the Boardwalk, Beach Club, or Yacht Club. Children can play on the beach by the Beach Club while waiting for their runner to pass by.

If your family wants to get in some park time during the race, Disney's Hollywood Studios and Epcot will open while the race is going on. Take a look at the course map to find where the race will run through the parks so you can stake out a spot to see your runner. Be sure to bring your park ticket as admission is required to enter these parks once the parks have been opened to the public.

A piece of advice: if you need to cross the course at any time, do so quickly as to not interrupt the runners' momentum.

The finish line is always a great place to watch your runner achieve their goal. This area can be extremely crowded, especially for those who do not purchase ChEAR Squad. Again, helium-filled balloons purchased the day before will help your runner spot you in the crowd.

Wine & Dine Half-Marathon

Since this is a nighttime race, spectator opportunities are quite limited. However, this race course does include multiple parks that give some great options near the end of the race.

Similar to the Walt Disney World Marathon, the runners exit Disney's Hollywood Studios to run toward the Boardwalk area and by the Yacht and Beach Club resorts. These are great locations at which to spot your runner and encourage them for their last mile. Keep in mind, you will not be able to make it to Epcot in time to see you runner finish.

The runners also run through Epcot, so the spectators that purchased a Finish Line Party ticket will be able to see their runner near The Land and Spaceship Earth. In fact, the spectators almost form a tunnel for the runners!

The finish line is open for spectators. Although there is not much room near the actual finish line, there are other locations throughout the last half- mile or so. Finish Line Party tickets are not required for this viewing location.

A reminder: race weekends bring more crowds, which means transportation will most likely be crowded and run slower than usual. Be sure to allow yourself plenty of time to get from one location to the next. Typical recommended travel time for Disney transportation is ninety minutes. With the increase in race weekend crowds, allow at least two hours of travel time.

Getting Around the Course

With road closures and runners, getting around the Walt Disney World Resort during a race can be tricky. It cannot be stressed enough, allow yourself plenty of time to get to your spectator location.

Host Resorts

It is highly recommended and encouraged that you stay at a host resort. With the road closures, this ensures that everyone is able to get to the race events on time.

If you are staying at a host resort, you can use the same race transportation as your runner, with runners getting priority. Keep in mind this means that you will also be at the race start a good two hours prior to the actual start of the event. From the family reunion area, you will need to find Disney transportation to the locations at which you are planning on watching your runner.

Morning Races

For the morning races, the monorail will begin running at 3 a.m. You can take the monorail from Epcot to the Transportation and Ticket Center then get on the monorail to Magic Kingdom. (You can then use this transportation back to Epcot for the finish.) It is highly encouraged you use the early transportation to the event before the start. There is only one entrance and exit into Epcot, which can get very congested after the race starts. You don't want to miss your runner!

For those staying at the Grand Floridian or Polynesian, you can sleep in a little and spot your runner along the service road behind the resorts. From there you can take the monorail to the Ticket and Transportation Center and on to Epcot for the finish.

Evening Races

For the evening races, normal park transportation will be available until park closing. Spectators should *not* use host resort race transportation with their runners since the race starts in different locations from where it ends.

Other Transportation Options

If you have a vehicle, you can park at any park's parking lot. Keep in mind that traffic may be hectic, especially with road closures, so you may miss a viewing location. Always plan enough time to make it to the finish line within your runner's finish time.

Taking a cab is a great idea for races that do not start at a park (like the Wine & Dine Half-Marathon). You can have your runner dropped off at the start line then have the cab bring you to your first viewing location.

ChEAR Squad

Looking for a way for your friends and family (who are not participating in a race) to get involved? Then the ChEAR Squad may be the answer. Available for the Walt Disney World Half-Marathon, Walt Disney World Marathon, Goofy's Race-and-a-Half Challenge, Dopey Challenge, and Princess Half-Marathon, your friends, family, guests, and other spectators can join in on the fun.

There are three packages to choose from. The first level is the Silver package, priced at $39. This includes a fun ChEAR Squad gear kit. This kit has a waterproof stadium blanket, Mickey clappers, and a ChEAR Squad t-shirt. At $39, the pricing isn't too bad for a shirt and blanket. However, if you aren't interested in either, skip this level. If you want prime seating locations, we recommend going with a higher level package.

The Gold package starts at $65. Along with the ChEAR Squad gear kit, you also get access to a reserved ChEAR Squad viewing location along the course. Also included is entrance to the ChEAR Squad Finish Line Zone, which includes reserved grandstand seating as well as beverages and private restrooms. (Viewing locations are first-come, first-serve.) This is a great option for spectators who are concerned about finding places to watch the race. The ChEAR Squad viewing locations are at Magic Kingdom (near Cinderella Castle) and at the finish line. Even better, children under the age of three can join you for free!

The ultimate ChEAR Squad experience is the Platinum package. Starting at $120, you get the ChEAR Squad gear kit, reserved viewing locations, and access to the Race Retreat. (See Chapter 11 for more information about the Race Retreat.) Race Retreat can be specifically advantageous for spectators with children under age three. A temperature-controlled environment with private restrooms and an area for the children to roam can be worth the extra cost. For some, the price of admission may be worth it not to have to worry about keeping the child entertained in the spectator stands while waiting for their runner to finish. Plus, Race Retreat is known to have a few characters stop by and provides an area for coloring or making support signs for the runner. Children who wish to zone out in the early morning hours will enjoy relaxing on comfy bean bag chairs while watching Disney movies. Another great advantage to the Platinum ChEAR Squad package is that children under age three are admitted to private areas, including Race Retreat, for free!

Pricing for Goofy's Race-and-a-Half Challenge and Dopey Challenge ChEAR Squad is slightly more than listed above.

The Gold or Platinum packages are a great way to ensure your family has great spectating locations along the race course. The Platinum option offers the Race Retreat, which can come in very handy if the weather is cool or rainy because the tent is climate controlled. This is a great option for the Walt Disney World Marathon as it offers a place to sit and eat before your runner finishes. However, if you have a particularly fast runner, the Platinum package may not offer you a lot of time to enjoy Race Retreat, except for after the race.

The Gold and Platinum viewing locations along Main Street USA are close to the castle, near the center hub by the Roy Disney and Mickey Mouse statue. From this location you will be able to see your runner coming down Main Street USA and turning into Tomorrowland. In theory, you should be able to go to the other side of the hub to see your runner come through Cinderella Castle. However, in past years, ChEAR Squad has been congested at times, meaning that it has not been possible to see your runner unless you arrive very early to secure a front row spot and then remain in place until your runner passes.

The ChEAR Squad grandstand seating at the finish line is located just before to the actual finish line. This allows for great finishing photos of your runner. These stands tend to be less congested, allowing for room to spread out and enjoy the wait at the finish. From these stands, you can see the runners coming out of Epcot, allowing you to spot your runner prior to the finish line. If you are worried about missing your runner at the finish, have them text or give you a call when they are in Future World, then keep an eye out for their outfit!

> I bought the gold level for my dad. He loved the gear, proudly wore his shirt and made use of the reserved bleachers at the finish. He enjoyed himself while waiting for my mom and me.
> *Sandi, AK*

What to Bring for Your Runner

Beyond being there to support your runner with your presence, camera, and support sign, you may want to bring a few more items for them. Having a small backpack or bag with some essentials such as water, fuel (gels, sport beans, fruit, pretzels, etc.), Band-Aids, BioFreeze, and extra socks would be a great idea. This way if something has happened along the course, your runner is covered. Prior to entering a park or the Family Reunion area, your bag will be checked by security.

Also, if your runner did not check a bag at the family reunion area, you may want to bring some items they may need after the race. A sweatshirt is a must as your runner may get chilled after the race. Any food or drink they may need can also be included.

What the Spectators Should Bring

It will be an early morning for you along with a lot of waiting as you look for your runner. Along with your camera, it is recommended you bring beverages and snacks. (See below for where to find these near the race course.) You will also want to bring your phone for runner tracking or if your runner calls you on the course. Don't forget your hat, sunglasses, and sunscreen for the sunny days, or a poncho and umbrella for the rainy days. Also, don't forget your park tickets/MagicBand if you will be entering a park after 9 a.m.

If you have kids in tow, you will want to bring entertainment for them. Toys, coloring books, iPad, or other options will keep them occupied while waiting for your runner. Other fun options are signs to hold up and candy to hand out to the runners.

For those going to the finish line area, you may want to bring a towel or blanket to sit on. If you are in the bleacher section, the seats may be cool or hot, so this saves your legs. If you are in a grassy area or parking lot, this allows a place to sit semi-comfortably.

Meeting Your Runner After the Race

You have watched your runner finish their big race. Now it's time to give them a big hug. There is a Family Reunion area available for you to meet at. This area has large signs with letters on it. Plan to meet at a specific letter (perhaps your last initial) so that you can find each other quickly. Having your cell phone would be a wise idea so that you can quickly contact each other in the sea of people.

Childcare During The Race

Need childcare during the race? All runDisney races do not allow strollers on the course. Therefore, parents of small children may need childcare during the race if both parents decide to run the same race. Kid's Nite Out provides sitter services to all Disney properties and is a preferred sitter service for the Walt Disney World resort. Sitter service may be arranged for twenty-four hours a day. Therefore, parents can rest assured that they will have a sitter at 3 a.m., if they need one. All sitters have full background checks and are fully CPR and first-aid certified. Sitters will arrive with games and activities to keep your children entertained while you are racing. Sitter services should be arranged in advance. There is also a minimum number of hours required for sitter services. For more information, contact Kid's Nite Out at **1-800-696-8105.**

Coffee, Snacks, and More

Spending several hours following your runner can work up an appetite! Where can you grab some food prior to park opening? If you are attending an after party, then you should not have any trouble finding food while waiting for your runner to cross the finish line. But what if you are following a runner during the early morning hours? As you leave Epcot, you will find coffee and pastries at the Transportation and Ticket Center near the area where you switch to the Magic Kingdom monorail. If the line is long, don't worry as there are other options available. Jump on the Magic Kingdom monorail and get off at the Polynesian Resort. Just inside the door of the Grand Ceremonial House, you will find the Kona Café serving coffee and pastries. You can also head downstairs to Captain Cook's for a quick breakfast. If neither of these stops fit into your schedule (You don't want to miss your runner.), coffee has previously been sold outside The Emporium on Main Street. If you need to use the restrooms, don't forget about the park restrooms as well as resort locations.

Krista & Megan's Tips

- Transportation runs slower during the race, so it is wise to get up with your runner. The lines (especially for the monorail) can get very long, and you don't want to miss your runner!

- When in doubt, get to the finish line. Don't try to squeeze in another viewing location by cutting it close. Get to the finish line to watch your runner cross.

- It can be awhile before you will see your runner, so make sure the little ones have items that will keep them occupied. (The big kids may need something too.)

- If you have small kids and you are following a runner, bring your own stroller. Stroller rental will not be available, and there is a lot of walking between transportation and viewing spots.

- Plan a location to meet your runner after the race. Whether in the parking lot, Family Reunion area near a certain letter sign, or someplace else, plan in advance. Sometimes cell service is spotty with so many cell phones in one location.

- When in doubt, pick a less crowded viewing spot on the course. You won't be able to get a good photograph of your runner in crowded viewing spots.

- In the past, there have been a few glitches with cell service due to the amount of people using phones during a race. Always have a back-up plan!

- If you have a runner participating in the Walt Disney World Marathon, the Platinum ChEAR Squad is an excellent option. Watch your runner at Magic Kingdom, then head back to Race Retreat for breakfast before watching your runner finish!

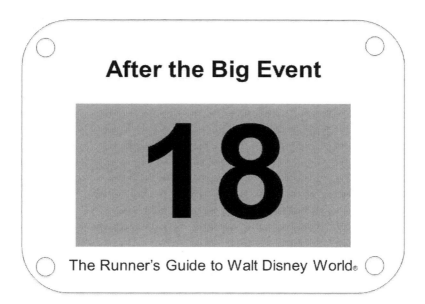

After the Big Event

The Runner's Guide to Walt Disney World®

Congratulations. You are officially a race finisher. Your legs may hurt. You may feel tired. You could eat an entire buffet. These are all normal feelings, so here are some suggestions on dealing with that tired body.

Recovery

Runners have many different tips to assist with recovery and avoid post-race soreness. Some popular tips include:

- Don't lie down. Although there is nothing you would rather do than take a long nap (especially if you had an early morning), do everything in your power to stay off the bed or couch.
- Take an ice bath or head into your resort pool. Although it's not comfortable, it does quicken your recovery time.
- Soak for at least twenty minutes in a warm bath of Epsom salts.
- Use compression gear. From pants to socks, this recovery tool can increase circulation and ease tired legs.
- Get something to eat. However, stick with foods you know will sit well. What have you had after your training runs?

Choose a restaurant that has similar foods and eat up. Even indulge a bit!

- Try Tart Cherry Juice. Studies have shown that drinking 6 oz. of Tart Cherry Juice twice a day seven days prior to the run and two days after can substantially reduce delayed muscle onset soreness.
- Keep hydrating. During your race, you most likely lost quite a bit of fluid. Make sure you keep drinking water and add in an electrolyte drink if it is particularly hot or humid outside.
- A great treat after your race is a massage at one of the Walt Disney World resort spas. This is a great way to get rid of the lactic acid in your muscles and a fun reward for your accomplishment. If your legs tend to be sore after a run, you may want to wait a day or two after the race when scheduling your massage.

Results

Immediately after the race, your results will be posted on the runDisney website. By clicking a link (that will take you to the **active.com** site), you can not only see your official finish time, but also other results. These include your placing among the other runners, as well as in your gender and age division. Feel free to gloat, or use it as motivation for your next race.

Photos

Did you smile for the camera? Were your arms raised high at the finish? How about that photo with your favorite character?

The photos from the race will be on **MarathonFOTO.com**. You should receive an email when these photos are available, usually a few days after the race. (It takes a while to look through thousands of photos.) You will then be able to look through the photos by race, then by your bib number or name.

In the past, it has taken a while for all of your photos to appear on the website. Be patient as more are uploaded throughout the days after the race. There may also be videos at various locations, depending on the race.

Did you find some photos you would like to purchase? Go for it. The photos aren't cheap, but some of the captured memories are worth the price. You can choose from digital photos (sent in an email), print photos, photo CDs, and even commemorative items. It is also wise to check their website a few weeks prior to the race, as they have included deals on gift cards or pre-purchases in the past.

Celebrations

After crossing the finish line, it will be time to celebrate. There are many great ways to celebrate your runDisney accomplishment throughout Walt Disney World Resort.

Behind the Scenes Tours

If you are a Disney enthusiast, a behind the scenes tour is a great way to celebrate your race achievement. Although it does mean more time on your feet, you will be able to experience the parks in a whole new way.

There are over 15 tours to choose from throughout the four theme parks. From the Behind the Seeds tour at The Land in Epcot to a VIP tour that covers all thrill rides, there is a tour for everyone. Most tours do have an age requirement (anywhere from 8 to 16 years of age), so your tour experience may be best with your spouse or friends.

A few unique tour options include:

Wild Africa Trek – Explore Harambe Reserve in a whole new way during this three-hour long tour. With the assistance of a harness, cross rope bridges and get up close and personal with a few exotic animals. A photographer will be there to capture the magical moments.

Keys to the Kingdom – Learn about the history of Walt Disney World Resort, along with Walt's philosophies and more during this five-hour tour. Experience backstage access, including a sneak peek at the underground village of Magic Kingdom. (For a longer experience, check out the Backstage Magic tour.)

Epcot DiveQuest – If you are a certified Scuba diver, this tour is for you. Dive into The Seas aquarium and swim with the tropical fish, sharks, stingrays and more. You may even be part of the entertainment for the Coral Reef restaurant goers!

Ultimate Day of Thrills – During race weekends, time is of the essence. During this tour, you will get to experience at least 10 of the major thrill rides at all four theme parks! The VIP treatment allows you to head to the front of the line. Tour is offered on limited days of the week. Call for availability.

VIP Tours – For the ultimate luxury experience, you can enjoy your very own VIP tour guide for a day in the parks. Not only will they offer information as you walk throughout the parks, they also will grant you FastPasses for most attractions! Your group can include up to 10 guests, making this pricey experience a little more reasonable. (Note: There is a 6-hour minimum for this tour and it needs to be booked in advance as it fills quickly.)

If you are interested in any of the behind the scenes tours, you can make your tour reservation 180 days before your arrival. Full payment is due at time of booking and those with Annual Passes, Disney Vacation Club or Disney Visa Cards may be able to get a small discount.

Fireworks Cruise

Looking for a new way to enjoy your favorite fireworks show? Taking a fireworks cruise may be just the ticket.

Set sail on the Grand 1 Yacht on Seven Seas Lagoon to watch Wishes from the water. This cruise can seat up to 18 guests and private dining can also be arranged.

For an unforgettable view, hop aboard the Breathless II to watch IllumiNations: Reflections of Earth. This boat anchors near the bridge between United Kingdom and France for a fabulous viewing. This boat can seat up to 6 guests and private dining can be arranged.

A cruise aboard a Sun Cruiser Pontoon boat is also available for both Magic Kingdom and Epcot fireworks shows. There is a 10 guest maximum and private dining is available.

Celebration Meal

After a race, it is very common for a runner to have one thing on their mind – food! A celebration meal is a great way to unwind from your race.

With over 200 restaurants throughout Walt Disney World Resort, there is something for everyone! To find the perfect restaurant to celebrate your accomplishment, check out Chapter 7.

Spa Treatment

After all the training and racing miles you have put in, it is time to relax! A great way to sit back and unwind is by enjoying one of the many fantastic spa treatments at Walt Disney World.

Health clubs are available at the following resorts: Disney's Animal Kingdom Lodge, Disney's Boardwalk Resort, Disney's Contemporary Resort, Disney's Coronado Springs Resort, Disney's Wilderness Lodge Resort and Disney's Yacht & Beach Club Resort. Each of these health clubs offers spa services such as massages, facials, manicures, pedicures and salon services.

If you are looking for a truly relaxing experience, then a trip to the Senses Spa is a must. Senses Spa is located at Disney's Grand Floridian Resort & Spa and Disney's Saratoga Springs Resort & Spa. Each treatment is based off of three experiences: Relax, Renew and Imagine. Along with various massage options, body treatments, manicures, pedicures and facials are available. Each treatment also includes various spa amenities.

Shopping

Sometimes a great race is followed with a little retail therapy. Throughout Walt Disney World Resort, there are many shopping locations. Each park includes various stores, however most carry similar items. Epcot and Animal Kingdom do have unique items, specifically in World Showcase and Africa, respectively.

Disney Springs also offers plenty of shopping, including new stores as Disney Springs continues to form. In the Marketplace, you can find various Disney-related items, from wine to art, kitchen to clothing. Head toward the West Side and you will find stores with less Disney, such as Curl by Sammy Duvall, Fit2Run, Something Silver, Harley-Davidson and more. In 2016, stores such as Zara, Tommy Bahama, Lilly Pulitzer and PANDORA will open as well.

Character Photos

Another unique aspect about racing in Walt Disney World is that you can get photos with characters while showing off that shiny new medal. In each park are various characters for you to get photos with. Take a look at the Times Guide (inside each park map at the park entrance or at your resort) or the My Disney Experience app to see what characters are around for you to get photos with.

You can also schedule FastPass+ for certain character photo opportunities as well. The most popular are Mickey and the gang, as well as Anna and Elsa from Frozen. If you want to secure any of these character experiences, be sure to make your FastPass+ reservations at your designated window. (See more in Chapter 19.) If you are a Disney Visa Rewards cardholder, there is a special character meet and greet just for you. Located in Innoventions West in Epcot, you can experience an exclusive event with two of the following characters: Mickey, Minnie, Goofy or Pluto. This is offered daily from 1 to 7 PM. All photos will be added to your MagicBand and/or Memory Maker package. However, if you stop by the image shop near the entrance of Epcot the same day, you receive a complimentary 5x7 photo from your meet and greet. Be sure to bring your Disney Visa card, as you will need to show it to the cast member at the meet and greet.

Finisher Certificate

A few weeks after the event, you will receive an email stating that your finisher certificate is available. These (along with other photos, videos and more) are available on **MyDisneyMarathon.com**.

What is a finisher certificate? It is themed for your event and lists your name and finish time and is even signed by important Disney personnel.

Some races do offer multiple certificates. For example, in the past, the Princess Half-Marathon offered certificate colors based on your favorite Disney princess. Feel free to print off more than one and hang them where you can see your accomplishment daily.

Post-Race Blues

You put in the training miles. You prepared for the event. You crossed the finish line. Now you may be feeling what is called post-race blues.

Do not be discouraged. Many runners go through this after a big race. Here are a few ideas on how to deal with the post-race (or even post-Disney) blues.

Create a scrapbook. Use race photos and vacation photos and create a scrapbook or photo book of your race and vacation. Include items such as your race bib, finisher certificate, and the like.

Display your bling. You worked hard to earn that beautiful medal, now show it off! Sport Hooks has fantastic Disney-inspired medal holders that will allow you to display your medals at home. They even have medal displays specific to the runDisney challenges and created the medal hanger for runDisney! Sport Hooks are at most runDisney Health and Fitness Expos and can also be found online at **HeavyMedalz.com**.

Write a race recap. Chronicle your race in writing. This will not only allow others to experience your race, but will also be a great item for you to look back and read.

Sign up for another race. Disney offers many great events, so don't be afraid to sign up for another. Maybe this one will be a night race. Or maybe you'll up the distance. The entertainment, medal, and magic will keep you coming back for more.

Krista & Megan's Tips

- During training, take note of what recovery works best and be sure to bring along any items you may need. (Options may be Epsom salts, compression socks, a foam roller, etc.)

- Give yourself an extra day after your race before heading home. Being cramped in an airplane or car is not ideal for those legs!

- After your accomplishment, a splurge is a great way to celebrate! Book a massage, fireworks cruise or special meal.

- Keep an eye on the website or social media accounts for MarathonFoto prior to the race weekend. They do offer deals on gift cards or photo packages from time to time.

- Even though you may be anxious to see photos from the race, give MarathonFoto a few days to sort all of the photos. It is recommended you don't purchase them until at least a week after the race to make sure you get them all.

- Wear your medal in the parks! It is very common to see the runners wearing their medal in the parks for a day or two. Not to mention, character photos with your medal are even more magical!

It's Not Just a Race, It's a Vacation Too

19

The Runner's Guide to Walt Disney World®

While at Walt Disney World for your runDisney race, you will want to visit the parks as well. Keep in mind that the weekend of the event will result in higher crowds due to the participants and their families. If you are able to stay a few days after the event, the crowds should thin out, resulting in smaller wait times in the parks. If this is not an option, don't worry. Below is some advice on making the most of your stay.

Tips for Touring Prior to the Race

If you plan extra days prior to the race start, then there are many steps you can take to make your visit more enjoyable. First, wear comfortable shoes that are broken in and can withstand park touring. The last thing any runner needs is blisters prior to the race.

Second, and this cannot be overstated, pace yourself. Plan for early morning park touring, then take a break mid-day to enjoy the resort pool followed by a leisurely dinner. The most important thing is to save your energy for race day. The average Walt Disney World park guest walks four to eight miles per day, and it is easy to get caught up in the excitement of the parks and exhaust your energy before you realize it.

A great new addition to visiting Walt Disney World theme parks is MyMagic+. By utilizing the My Disney Experience app, you will be able to secure three FastPass+ selections each day. Our personal opinion is that MyMagic+ improves runner's touring experience and will make staying on property more important than ever. Prior to MyMagic+, race participants had to arrive at a park and pick up a FastPass to enjoy popular attractions without waiting in line. Arriving at a park in time to secure a FastPass for some of your favorite rides would often prove impossible. With MagicBands and FastPass+, race participants and family members will be able to schedule their favorite FastPass attractions at the park of their choice prior to the start of their vacation. Currently, FastPass+ allows guests to select up to three attractions per day, and you can schedule your ride times in advance. Once you use your three FastPass+ selections, you can then visit a kiosk inside the park to schedule another FastPass+, even in a different park.

If you are planning to tour prior to the race, keep in mind that some rides may not be tolerated well. If you are prone to motion sickness, then save the thrill rides for post-race.

Some rides that may induce motion sickness include:

Magic Kingdom
- Mad Tea Party
- Big Thunder Mountain
- Space Mountain

Epcot
- Mission: Space

Hollywood Studios
- Star Tours
- Rock 'N' Roller Coaster
- The Twilight Zone Tower of Terror

Animal Kingdom
- Expedition Everest
- Dinosaur

Tips for Touring After the Race

Touring after the race? If you are participating in a morning race, one of the benefits of an extremely early morning start time is finishing with plenty of time to take a nap and still enjoy an afternoon or evening at the parks. With FastPass+, you can schedule your attractions for later in the day, bypassing the lines.

Post-race touring allows time to focus on two separate events: the race followed by recovery and dedicated park time. This is the best plan for those who can accommodate this schedule into their vacation plans.

FastPass+

FastPass+ (*FP+*) allows you to skip the line and go directly to the ride. Usual wait time using FastPass+ is less than five minutes. FastPasses are complimentary. These are scheduled ahead of time (for those staying at a Disney resort or who have a MagicBand) as well as inside the park at a FP+ kiosk. You will need FastPass+ for each person over three years of age. (Kids under three will be allowed to ride with a guardian without FastPass+.) All FastPasses are coded to your MagicBand or park ticket.

FastPass+ selections can be made 60 days before arrival for those staying at a Disney resort. For guests staying off property, selections can be made 30 days prior to arrival. All guests are able to use the kiosks inside the park to make or adjust FastPass+

selections, as well as the My Disney Experience app on your smartphone.

When making your FP+ selections, each park is slightly different. For Magic Kingdom and Animal Kingdom, you are able to choose three attractions from throughout the park. For Epcot and Hollywood Studios, you choose one attraction from the first tier or group (the more popular attractions), and then two from the rest of the attractions in the park. Certain character meet-and-greets, along with parade and firework viewings, are also selections for FastPass+.

The FastPass+ has a time window that will tell you when to come back and ride. This is located in your My Disney Experience app. For example, your FastPass may indicate your return window is 10:35-11:35 a.m. You cannot ride before 10:35 a.m. and you *must* arrive in line by 11:35 a.m. Ending times are now strictly enforced, which is a recent change in the Disney FastPass system.

After using your three scheduled FastPass+ selections (all at the same park), you can then go to a FP+ kiosk inside any park to schedule another one. Once you use the fourth, you can then head back to the kiosk for a fifth, and so on. The first three must be in the same park, however any after that can be in a different park.

One thing to consider when making your original FP+ selections is whether you would like to use more than three FP+ or if you would like to use them for the parades and fireworks. If you wait to use one of your original three FP+ selections for a reserved viewing of the fireworks, you will not be able to visit a kiosk to select more than your original three selections.

Didn't get the FastPass+ reservation you wanted? Keep checking the website or your app for availability. It may suddenly appear, even while you are in the park.

What to See and When to See It

You are ready to head to the parks, so you may be wondering what must-do attractions you should see first. Here are some tips to get you headed in the right direction.

Virtually every attraction within all four theme parks uses FP+, however each park has rides that are considered major attractions. These rides usually have the longest wait times since they are the most popular. Consider using FastPass+ (see above) to reduce your wait times.

Major Attractions at Each Park

Magic Kingdom

Tomorrowland

Space Mountain - This roller coaster in the dark will send you on a space voyage you won't soon forget.

Buzz Lightyear's Space Ranger Spin - Use your sharp-shooting skills to defeat Zurg on this family-friendly ride.

Fantasyland

Dumbo the Flying Elephant - This Disney classic is not to be missed by those who are young or young at heart.

Seven Dwarfs Mine Train – The newest attraction at Magic Kingdom is a coaster-type trip through the jewel mines with your favorite dwarfs.

Peter Pan's Flight - Fly along with Peter Pan and Tinker Bell as you enjoy this classic ride with aerial views of London and Neverland.

It's a Small World - Enjoy a leisurely boat ride through various countries as dolls sing the classic "It's a Small World."

Under the Sea: Journey with the Little Mermaid – Join Ariel on her Under the Sea adventure.

Liberty Square

Haunted Mansion - Join 999 happy haunts on this ride in the dark through the Haunted Mansion.

Hall of Presidents - Widescreen film details the history of the United States followed by a roll call of every U.S. president portrayed in realistic audio-animatronic form.

Adventureland

Pirates of the Caribbean - Sail through the Spanish Main as you join Captain Jack Sparrow on this pirate adventure.

Jungle Cruise - An outdoor boat ride filled with adventure and laughs.

Frontierland

Big Thunder Mountain Railroad - Head to a mining town in the west on this roller coaster that is filled with twists and turns.

Splash Mountain – This log ride tells the classic tale of Br'er Rabbit. Final drop is fifty-two feet.

Epcot

Future World

Soarin' - Soar along on this simulated hang glider through the beautiful landmarks of California.

Test Track - Jump in your vehicle to put your car through its paces as you journey along on the test track, which involves a safety course and a high-speed run.

Mission: Space - Strap in for a space launch to Mars. Two versions of the ride are available with one version that spins for realistic simulation and one that does not.

Spaceship Earth - Audio-animatronic scenes detail this history of communication on this ride that is inside the Epcot ball.

Hollywood Studios

Hollywood Studios is undergoing a major refurbishment as the additions of Star Wars Land and Toy Story Land are being built. Keep in mind that this may affect portions of this park and adjust your plans accordingly.

Toy Story Midway Mania - A 4D ride that is fun for the whole family. Get ready to join Woody, Buzz, and your favorite *Toy Story* characters as you engage in a fun-filled arcade-style game.

Rock 'N' Roller Coaster - Join Aerosmith for twists and turns (and even an inversion or two) on this high-speed coaster in the dark.

The Twilight Zone Tower of Terror - Enjoy the detail starting with the walk up to the attraction on this free-falling thrill ride that beckons you to check in to the Hollywood Tower Hotel.

Star Tours - Exciting whirlwind 3D tour through the major planets and movie scenes of the Star Wars universe. With over fifty different worlds, each ride is different.

Animal Kingdom

Expedition Everest - Climb Everest via an exciting coaster to find the Yeti on this thrill-ride that features an eighty-foot drop and twists and turns that are both forward and backward.

Kilimanjaro Safaris - Encounter live animals on safari as you ride in an open-air vehicle through the savannah with your tour guide, looking for elephants, giraffes, lions, crocodiles, and other creatures of the wild.

Dinosaur - Head back in time to search for dinosaurs on this thrill ride that invokes a jerky but fun-filled adventure.

Character Meet-and-Greets

Throughout the parks are various opportunities to meet your favorite Disney characters. Be sure to look over the Times Guide (located in your park map) or through the My Disney Experience app for the times and locations of each character opportunity. Make sure you are equipped with an autograph book and pen to collect a signature to accompany the photograph with you and your favorite Disney characters. Autograph books are available throughout the parks and resorts.

Certain character meet-and-greets are also an option for FastPass+. Without a doubt, the most popular characters are Anna and Elsa in Magic Kingdom. Obtaining FastPass+ can be difficult, however it will reduce your wait time in line dramatically if you are able to grab one.

Parades and Fireworks

In true Disney magic, every day includes shows, parades, and nighttime spectaculars for your family to enjoy. FastPass+ selections are available for each parade and firework show, allowing your family to enjoy a reserved area to view the magic. Be sure to check the Times Guide or the My Disney Experience app for the official show times.

Magic Kingdom

Festival of Fantasy Parade, 3 p.m. – The newest parade at Walt Disney World is a celebration of your favorite Disney stories with a Fantasyland flair. Be on the lookout for your favorite Disney characters (including many princesses) as well as Maleficent as a fire-breathing dragon.

Main Street Electrical Parade, an hour before park closing - Watch the bright lights of the floats, along with your favorite characters, in this nighttime parade. Check the schedule when you arrive as this parade may not occur every night of the week.

Wishes, at park closing - Fireworks and music help make your favorite Disney dreams come true! Jiminy Cricket narrates a historical tour of classic Disney moments.

Epcot

Illuminations, 9 p.m. - Watch as World Showcase Lagoon is transformed with lasers, fireworks, fountains, and more. Even the countries around World Showcase get in on the fun.

Hollywood Studios

Fantasmic!, around park closing - This twenty-five-minute fireworks and water show follows Sorcerer Mickey along with many familiar characters. Your favorite Disney songs and video clips are also involved.

Water Parks

Along with the four theme parks, Walt Disney World also includes two water parks. Access to the water parks is through a separate ticket, or the addition of the water park option to your theme park tickets.

For runners staying a few days after the race, this is a great way to relax while still enjoying the feel of a theme park. However, due to walking up stairs and the possibility of sunburn, it may not be the best idea before a big race.

At Typhoon Lagoon, take off on various waterslides, a children's play area, a wave pool and lazy river. For an unforgettable experience, head to the Shark Reef where you will snorkel with sharks, stingrays and schools of fish. There is even a surf school where you can ride the waves!

A ski resort is beginning to melt away at Blizzard Beach. Along with waterslides, lazy river and wave pool, there is also a great play area for kids. Get the entire family on Teamboat Springs as you ride your raft down a waterslide. There is even an option to race each other on a toboggan.

Updates to the Parks

There are two major updates occurring at this time at the theme parks in Walt Disney World. In Animal Kingdom, Pandora: The World of Avatar is in the building process. This new addition is expected to open in 2017.

Hollywood Studios is also in the midst of a major refurbishment. Star Wars Land and Toy Story Land have been announced for this park. No opening dates have been set, however this may impact areas of the park, so adjust your plans accordingly.

Along with these large updates, there are times when attractions undergo refurbishments as well. Visit **http://disneyworld.disney.go.com/wdw/** to stay up-to-date on any closings of attractions.

Sights Outside the Parks

Perhaps you will only be visiting Walt Disney World for a short period of time, or maybe you would like to try something beyond the parks. Here are some great options of things to see outside of the theme parks.

Resorts

Each Walt Disney World resort has its own special theme. Taking the time to explore resorts other than your own is a great idea for an afternoon. Take the monorail to the three monorail resorts. Hop on a bus to a resort you have never experienced. Make a dining reservation at a resort restaurant you've been meaning to try. Then explore.

Disney Springs

Disney Springs is currently transforming into Disney Springs. Construction is well underway, which means there may be limited parking and many walls up around certain areas. Once complete (sometime in 2016), Disney Springs will include more than 150 shopping, dining and entertainment venues, as well as a large parking structure.

This shopping and entertainment district is a great option as no park ticket is required. Shop until you drop at stores such as Once Upon a Toy, Disney's Days of Christmas, World of Disney, D Street, Basin, and many others. Be sure to take in some of the great restaurants as well, especially Ghirardelli for a post-race treat.

Stop by Splitsville and participate in one of America's favorite past-times. This luxury bowling alley and dinner lounge offers 45,000 square feet of fun and entertainment. With thirty bowling lanes, patio dining, and live music spread over two floors, Splitsville will provide hours of entertainment for the entire family.

Perhaps you would just like to take it easy before (or after) your race. The AMC movie theater offers the latest movies for your family to enjoy. You can even partake in the dine-in experience and have dinner while watching the movie.

If you are looking for a unique nighttime activity, get tickets for Cirque du Soleil - La Nouba. This show is a family favorite as acrobats take the stage in fun ways.

As the transformation into Disney Springs continues, another change is to Disney Quest. In 2016, Disney Quest will close and will make way for the new NBA Experience.

Special Events

Throughout the year, Disney has special events that are favorites among many. Here are a few of the fun events your family can enjoy during race weekends.

Epcot's Flower and Garden Festival - From the beginning of March through mid-May, Epcot's landscaping gets a boost for the Flower and Garden Festival. See your favorite Disney characters brought to life through beautiful topiaries and flower sculptures. You can even head into a butterfly house. (The festival is included with park admission.) The Flower and Garden Festival occurs during Star Wars Half Marathon Weekend – The Dark Side.

Mickey's Not-So-Scary Halloween Party - From the beginning of September through the beginning of November, Magic Kingdom hosts a special evening Halloween party. Dress up and trick-or-treat with your favorite Disney characters. Enjoy the attractions, and even watch a special parade and fireworks show. This is a separate ticketed event beginning at $68 per adult and $63 per child aged three to nine.

Epcot's International Food and Wine Festival - From the end of September through mid-November, Epcot hosts the largest Food and Wine Festival in the United States. Food carts from around the world emerge in the World Showcase, allowing you to experience food and wine from many countries. You can even enroll in special culinary or wine tasting classes. (Some classes are an additional cost.) Be careful not to partake in too much prior to your race, but afterward feel free to celebrate. (The Festival is included with park admission.) The Food and Wine Festival occurs during the Wine & Dine Half-Marathon.

Mickey's Very Merry Christmas Party - From the beginning of November through the end of December, Magic Kingdom hosts a great evening Christmas party. Along with experiencing your favorite attractions and character meet-and-greets, watch the Christmas parade and fireworks show. You can even watch Cinderella's Castle transform into a beautiful lighted spectacle. This is a separate ticketed event beginning at $74 per adult and $69 per child aged three to nine. The Christmas Party is an option for those participating the Wine & Dine Half-Marathon.

In the months leading up to your vacation, be sure to check if new special events are occurring during your stay. It has been very common for Disney to announce fun (ticketed) events like dessert parties during the nighttime shows, exclusive morning tours and much more.

Krista & Megan's Tips

- Stay on property so that you can utilize Magic Bands and FastPass+ to schedule attractions on race day.

- Save rides that might induce motion-sickness for after the race.

- Pace yourself! You don't want to expend you energy at the parks prior to race day.

- Touring pre-race? Pick a theme park with less ground to cover than one of the larger parks. Good choices include Hollywood Studios or focus on one or two areas in Magic Kingdom.

- If you are participating during the Wine & Dine Half Marathon Weekend, be sure to experience Mickey's Very Merry Christmas Party. This is a great way to experience a little extra Disney magic.

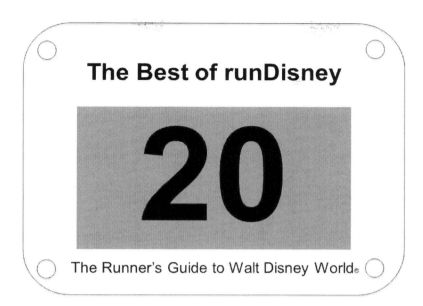

The Best of runDisney

20

The Runner's Guide to Walt Disney World®

Many runners who are new to runDisney want to know, where is the best place to eat? What is the best race to run? Where is the best place to stay? While these answers depend on many factors, here is a "Best of runDisney" section to help guide you along the way.

Best runDisney Race for Beginners

Princess Half-Marathon Weekend
(also Wine & Dine Half-Marathon Weekend)

When trying to choose the best race weekend as your first race, there are many options. Many choose based on a theme. Others choose on a race distance. When it comes to beginners, Princess Half-Marathon Weekend offers a great experience. Many others choose this as their first, primarily due to the theme, meaning you will not be the only beginner. It offers a variety of race distances as well as decent weather due to the late February date.

Another great weekend is Wine & Dine Half-Marathon Weekend. The 5K is one of the best, which is a great option for beginning runners. This race weekend also follows a theme that anyone can enjoy (whereas some men may not be so keen on the princess theme).

Best runDisney 5K

Jingle Jungle 5K

Mickey's Jingle Jungle 5K during Wine & Dine Half-Marathon Weekend is one of the best 5K races runDisney offers. Along with a unique race course that takes you through Animal Kingdom theme park, you also will experience characters in their holiday best. Not to mention, this race includes one of the latest morning start times.

Best runDisney 10K

Walt Disney World 10K

Since both 10K races cover the same course, it can be hard to choose a best race. One advantage the Walt Disney World 10K has is (possibly) cooler weather.

*Note: Once the course is confirmed, it is very possible that the Star Wars 10K – The Dark Side will take over this category!

Best runDisney Half-Marathon

Wine & Dine Half-Marathon

As the only half-marathon to cover three parks, the Wine & Dine Half-Marathon is a fan favorite. While the night race aspect can be hard to prepare for, the entertainment is spectacular throughout this course. Running through the Osborne Family Spectacle of Dancing Lights is something you are sure to remember forever, not to mention partying until 4 a.m. after the race.

Best runDisney Challenge

Goofy's Race-and-a-Half Challenge (also The Dark Side Challenge)

The runDisney challenges are definitely on the rise, but how do you choose which one to tackle? For those with running experience (it is recommended to have a marathon under your belt), Goofy's Race-and-a-Half Challenge is a great option. The January event is the largest and brings out a crowd. Along with the half-marathon, run through all four theme parks and ESPN Wide World of Sports during the marathon on the second day.

If you don't have quite as much running experience (or don't want to tackle 39.3 miles), the Dark Side Challenge will be another fun option. With some of the best theming throughout the weekend, you can earn that third medal in style.

Best runDisney Race Weather

Wine & Dine Half-Marathon Weekend

It's no secret that Florida can have some crazy weather. While race day conditions cannot be predicted, history shows that the November Wine & Dine Half-Marathon Weekend seems to have the best overall experience. Expect temperatures in the 60s or 70s along with lower humidity. (If you are from northern areas, note that this still will seem warm to you.)

Best runDisney Race Theme

Princess Half-Marathon Weekend
(also Star Wars Half-Marathon Weekend – The Dark Side)

One aspect that has been taking over runDisney race weekends are themes. When it comes to the Walt Disney World races, Princess

Half-Marathon Weekend is a winner. There is no doubt that you will feel like royalty from the red carpet at the Expo to the cheers at the finish.

With the addition of a Star Wars race on the west coast, there is no question that this will be another well-themed race weekend. From your favorite Star Wars characters to fantastic costumes, this is sure to be a fan favorite.

Best Walt Disney World Resort Hotels (based by runDisney Race Weekend)

Walt Disney World Marathon Weekend/Princess Half-Marathon Weekend

Monorail Resorts – Disney's Grand Floridian Resort & Spa, Disney's Polynesian Village Resort or Disney's Contemporary Resort

When it comes to convenience during these race weekends, the monorail resorts cannot be beat. On race morning, runners can take the monorail to Epcot, then walk to the race start area. For the longer races, spectators can take the monorail to Magic Kingdom, or they can take a short walk to spectate along the service road.

Star Wars Half-Marathon Weekend

While the host resorts and courses for this weekend have not yet been determined, it does appear that Epcot and ESPN Wide World of Sports Complex will be included in the weekend races. For that reason, the Epcot Resorts – Disney's Boardwalk Inn, Disney's Beach Club Resort or Disney's Yacht Club Resort are great options. Disney's Art of Animation is also another resort to consider as it will be a short bus ride after the race is done.

Epcot Resorts – Disney's Boardwalk Inn, Disney's Beach Club Resort or Disney's Yacht Club Resort

With a race that includes a fun after-party in Epcot, being able to walk back to your resort is definitely a great option. (You will have to take a bus to the start.) Spectators will also have a great view as you come through the Epcot resort area. From there, they can join you at the Finish Line Party (with a party ticket) or head back to the resort to sleep.

Best Value Resort

Disney's Art of Animation Resort (also Disney's Pop Century Resort)

As Walt Disney World's newest resort, this is hands-down the best value resort. Enjoy standard rooms with a Little Mermaid theme, or spend a little more for the family suites that include a dedicated master bedroom, mini-kitchen and an extra bathroom. Along with great theming and pools, the food court is one of the best on Disney property.

Deciding between the other value resorts? Disney's Pop Century is definitely the one to choose. With only one bus stop, it will save you a lot of time off the bus and in the parks and along with Art of Animation, Pop Century one of the best food courts on Disney property.

Best Moderate Resort

Disney's Port Orleans Resort - Riverside

When it comes to the moderate resorts, the relaxing atmosphere of Disney's Port Orleans Resort is just what a runner needs. The buildings are not spread out like the other resorts, meaning less time on your feet before a race.

Best Deluxe Resort

Disney's Animal Kingdom Lodge

While all of the deluxe resorts offer fantastic amenities, proximity to the parks and theme, the unique atmosphere and design of Disney's Animal Kingdom Lodge is superb. Where else (except in Africa) can you look out your balcony and see giraffes, zebras and other exotic wildlife? Not to mention, the lobby is beautiful and the cast members are eager to answer questions about their culture.

Best Monorail Resort

Disney's Polynesian Village Resort

Staying along the monorail is an experience that many dream of. Disney's Polynesian Village not only offers monorail transportation, but also includes a theme that makes you feel you have stepped into the Pacific islands. With great restaurant options and a volcano-themed pool, it is a getaway to remember. (Note: Construction continues through early 2016.)

Best Epcot Resort

Disney's Beach Club Resort

The convenience of walking to Epcot (and even Hollywood Studios) is a fantastic option, especially for dining reservations. Add in the best pool on Disney property and Disney's Beach Club Resort is a must. It also is a great spectating location for the Walt Disney World Marathon and Wine & Dine Half-Marathon. Why does Beach Club edge out their sister resort, Yacht Club? Simply because Yacht

Club does not have a quick service restaurant. And, the short walk to Beach Club can be quite long for a quick meal post-race.

Best Resort for a Group

Disney's Art of Animation (also Disney's Saratoga Springs Resort)

For some participants, race weekends mean time with friends and family. If you want to all stay together, there are many options to do so. Suites may be out of the price range, so Disney's Art of Animation offers smaller family suites with a more manageable price tag.

If you would like something larger, the Deluxe Villa Resorts offer multiple bedroom options, including a full kitchen. Disney's Saratoga Springs is a great way for up to 9 people to stay together and offers easy access to Disney Springs for numerous dining options.

Best Pre-Race Meal

Via Napoli

Runners love to carb-load before a big race. While there are plenty of pasta options (both table service and quick service) throughout Walt Disney World, a favorite is Via Napoli in Epcot. This authentic Italian restaurant offers pizza and pasta to keep runners energized for their upcoming race. (For those with food allergies, gluten-free pasta is available at this location.)

Best Celebration Meal (based on meal type)

Dinner Show

Hoop Dee Doo Musical Revue

A dinner show is a great way to celebrate your runDisney race. With three to choose from, the Hoop Dee Doo Musical Revue is a must. Unlimited beer and sangria and a show that will keep you laughing is a perfect way to celebrate your race accomplishments.

Signature Meal

California Grill

For those wanting a nicer meal to celebrate, there are various signature meals throughout Walt Disney World. The newly refurbished California Grill is a neat option. Along with fantastic food, you get a bird's eye view of Cinderella Castle. Time it correctly and you can watch Wishes from above.

Character Meal

Cinderella's Royal Table (also Tusker House)

If you want to celebrate with your favorite characters, Cinderella's Royal Table is a truly unique experience. Join your favorite princesses in Cinderella Castle.

If you are looking for a great meal with Mickey and friends, try Tusker House at Animal Kingdom. This location has characters for breakfast and lunch and the food quality is far superior to Chef Mickey's.

Best Table Service Restaurant (based by park or resort)

Magic Kingdom

Be Our Guest

Transport yourself to the Beast's castle, where you can dine in the grand ballroom or visit the West Wing. Be sure to try the grey stuff, we hear it's delicious.

Epcot

World Showcase Restaurants

While it is difficult to choose just one, World Showcase offers many unique restaurants to enjoy. Feeling like Mexican? Head to San Angel Inn for a romantic dinner. Want to have fun? Go to Germany for the Biergarten hoopla. It may take a few race weekends to experience them all.

Hollywood Studios

50's Prime Time

Dine in mom's kitchen as you head back to the 50's for a hearty meal at 50's Prime Time – make sure you use your manners and don't put your elbows on the table.

Animal Kingdom

Tusker House

This buffet-style meal allows you to experience a taste of Africa. If you schedule a breakfast or lunch, you'll even get visits from Donald, Mickey, Goofy and Daisy.

Disney Springs

Portobello

This Italian restaurant is another great location to carb-load before a race. You can choose from various pizza and pasta options. If the weather is right, ask for a seat outside to get a glimpse of the Disney Springs excitement.

Walt Disney World Resort hotels

The Wave

Looking for one of the best hidden gems of Walt Disney World? Check out The Wave! No doubt Boma, 'Ohana and many other resort restaurants and excellent and extremely popular. However, for a seasonally-inspired menu that offers healthy options along with several decadent treats, you won't go wrong with The Wave.

Best Counter Service Restaurant (based by park or resort)

Magic Kingdom

Be Our Guest (also Columbia Harbour House)

Hands-down one of the most popular restaurants in Magic Kingdom, Be Our Guest is a favorite for lunch. The lines to get in tend to be long (unless you are able to get an elusive Fastpass+), so plan accordingly.

Since Be Our Guest can be difficult to get into, another favorite is Columbia Harbour House. There are multiple salads and sandwiches to choose from. You can even get away from the hustle and bustle by finding a seat upstairs.

Epcot

Sunshine Seasons

With options like soups, salads, stir fry and rotisserie chicken, there is something for everyone at this food court-style restaurant. You can even plan a ride on Soarin' before your meal.

Hollywood Studios

Pizza Planet (also Starring Rolls)

Head inside the pizzeria made famous in Toy Story. While the options are limited, there are arcade style games to keep you entertained.

Looking for a less greasy option? Starring Rolls has giant sandwiches that are sure to please the appetite. (Be sure to save room for one of the giant cupcakes as well.)

Animal Kingdom

Flame Tree BBQ

Take a break from the wildlife and enjoy ribs, chicken and sandwiches at Flame Tree BBQ.

Disney Springs

Earl of Sandwich

A favorite at Disney Springs is Earl of Sandwich. With a great menu full of unique sandwiches and salads, you are sure to find something that will please your taste buds. (If you go during the holidays, be sure to check out the holiday sandwich.)

Walt Disney World Resort hotels

Landscape of Flavors (Disney's Art of Animation Resort)

Create-your-own specialties at one of the best food courts on Disney property. Pasta, pizza, sandwiches, the possibilities are endless.

No matter what race weekend, resort or restaurant you choose, you are sure to experience many magical miles during your runDisney race weekend at Walt Disney World!

Appendix

A. Frequently Asked Questions

Accommodations

Are there any race registration discounts?
Race discounts are no longer available.

Are there discounts at Disney resorts for race participants?
Yes, there are. The host resorts often have discounts for race participants and discounted tickets and dining plan pricing. Check with your Authorized Disney Vacation Planner regarding these discounts (or other packages they may have available).

Can you bring your own food to the hotel? Do all the Walt Disney World hotels have refrigerators?
You can absolutely bring your own food to any Walt Disney World Resort hotel. There are various online grocery stores that will deliver food to Bell Services at your resort (for a fee). All Walt Disney World Resort hotels have a mini-fridge, with the 1-Bedroom and 2-Bedroom Villas having a full size refrigerator.

Which hotels offer race transportation?
During the Walt Disney World Marathon Weekend and Princess Half Marathon Weekend events, all Walt Disney World Resort hotels will offer race transportation. During the other race weekends, check runDisney.com to see what hotels are considered host resorts.

I'm not ready for a longer distance race yet, but I will be participating in the 5K. Does the expo and transportation information still apply to me?
Absolutely. If you are staying at a host resort, transportation will be provided to the expo and 5K event. We still advise that you arrive to the 5K early so that you have time to use the restroom and line up prior to the race. (Transportation usually stops an hour before the event.)

Pre-Race

Where are the best places to eat prior to a runDisney race?
Ultimately, it will depend on what type of food you normally eat before a long run or race. With hundreds of restaurants on Walt Disney World property, there are many to choose from. See Chapter 7 for information on all the restaurants, including a few pre-race favorites.

Can non-runners purchase the race extras such as Race Retreat, Pasta in the Park Party, Post-Race Breakfast, etc.?
Spectators, friends and family can absolutely purchase the race extras. The only one that is a little different is Race Retreat. Instead of purchasing Race Retreat, non-runners will need to purchase the Platinum ChEAR Squad instead. This will grant them access to spectating locations in Magic Kingdom and at the finish line, along with Race Retreat perks once the race has started.

If driving to a race start, how early should we arrive? What is the latest we can arrive?
Most traffic will begin around 3 a.m. through approximately 4:30 a.m. It is always advised to err on the side of caution and allow yourself extra time in case there is any traffic congestion. (Keep in mind, there is only one entrance into Epcot.) It is recommended to get to the Epcot parking lots no later than 4:30 a.m. as the walk to the Family Reunion area followed by the walk to the starting corrals is quite long.

What food is available pre-race?
Many Walt Disney World Resort hotels will have a quick service restaurant open for runners before the morning races. (It is highly recommended you check with your hotel prior to race morning.) There also has been a "runner's box" for purchase the day before races as well. At the Family Reunion area near the start, there are concession stands available.

What is the best way to fuel for a night race?
In our experience, it is best to eat your larger meal at lunch, followed by a smaller and easily digestible dinner. In the hour or two before the race, fuel as you would for any training run or race.

Where is the bus stop at the host resorts for race transportation?

The bus stops are located outside of the lobby area. There are Runner Transportation signs that will direct you. If you have any questions, ask a cast member.

Can our family take race transportation with us?
Yes they can and it is highly recommended for the morning races (as road closures will make transportation slower once the race starts). However, priority is given to runners.

When I registered for my race, I did not have a previous race qualifying time or I have since completed a race with a time that I think would allow me to improve my corral placement. How can I submit my time or improve my corral placement?
If it is more than two months before the race, you can submit your new race time by filling out the form on runDisney's website. Go to the race you want to update and look for Proof of Time under Runner Info. As a reminder, you cannot bring a proof of time to the Expo to change your corral.

During the Race

What type of sports drink and fuel is offered on the race course?
For the 5K and 10K races, only water is offered at the aid stations. For races of half-marathon length or longer, Powerade is offered as well as at least one fuel station. On the half marathon courses, Clif Shot gels are given around mile 9. On the marathon course, Clif Shot gels are available around miles 9, 16 and 19, bananas around miles 14 and 19, and chocolate around mile 23.

Where are the bathrooms on the course?
Port-o-potties are located along the course, including the start, finish and near the aid stations. If your race course includes a park, be sure to take advantage of the "real" bathrooms.

If I'm injured/sick during the race, will I still get a medal?
While there is no official answer to this question, it is rumored that those who do not finish still get a medal. This is always subject to change as the runDisney website does state it is a finisher's medal.

Do the races ever get cancelled due to weather?
runDisney events occur rain or shine, cold or hot. The only exception is lightning. If that is the case, the event may have a delayed start or be cancelled. This will be determined by event staff and communicated with the participants.

Will roads be closed for the race?
Yes, the roads that you run on during the longer events are closed to vehicles to ensure the safety of the runners. These are outlined in your final race instructions, so plan your driving route accordingly and be sure to allow yourself plenty of time to get to the start if you are driving. This is one of the reasons it is highly encouraged you stay at a host resort and use race transportation.

I am running with a friend who was placed in a faster corral. Can we run together?
Yes. Runners placed in a faster corral may move back with no issues. For example, a runner who is placed in corral B can run with a friend in corral D and will be allowed to enter corral D at the race start. Corral D runner cannot move up and will not be allowed to enter corral B.

As a runner, do I need a park ticket for the race itself? Do we get park tickets for the day after the race?
You do not need a park ticket for your race. (Can you imagine the congestion at the turnstiles trying to get your ticket scanned?) Unfortunately, runners are no longer given park tickets or free admission on the day after a race. You can purchase discounted tickets through runDisney.

Do spectators need a park ticket to watch their runners inside the parks?
To watch your runner along Main Street USA in Magic Kingdom at Walt Disney World, you will not need a theme park ticket. However, to watch your runner in any other park, you will (as the park will then be open to the public). The finish lines are all located outside of the parks, so you can still watch your runner finish.

If I am staying at an Epcot resort, can I walk to the start of my race?
For the Walt Disney World Marathon Weekend and Princess Half-Marathon Weekend events, no. For the Wine & Dine Half-Marathon, yes with proper park tickets. (Keep in mind that for the Wine & Dine Half-Marathon, the race begins at ESPN Wide World of Sports. Therefore, spectators can walk through Epcot to the finish area in the parking lot prior to park closing at 9 pm.)

I am running one of the night events. Can I leave the party to take a quick shower or change and then return to the party?
There are two options. The first is that there will be changing areas available, so you can put a change of clothes in your bag check, and then change at the party. (There are lockers available for rent to store your bag.) If you choose to go back to your resort, be certain to bring your after party wristband to the party as that will be your entrance "ticket."

After the Race

What food is available after the race?
Directly after the race, runners enter the finisher's chute where bananas and a box with various food is available. In the past, the box has included crackers, fruit snacks, etc. There are also concessions available in the Family Reunion area. If the parks are open, you can visit the restaurants there or head back to your resort for a meal.

Are there washing/showering facilities after the race?
Changing tents are available, however showering facilities are not.

If I run the 5K, do I get an entry into the after parties?
Unfortunately, the automatic entry is for those participating in the longer distance events. (The only exception is for the Walt Disney World Marathon Weekend and Princess Half-Marathon Weekend as those after parties are free to all.) You can purchase tickets to the Wine & Dine Finish Line Party on the runDisney website.

Misc.

For those who aren't used to running in the (potential) Florida heat, what advice would you offer?
Florida weather can be unpredictable. If you are coming from a more northern climate, the potential heat and humidity can be a fear. Try to get in a few training runs on the treadmill, where the gym or house offer more heat. On race day, it is wise to slow down if it is exceptionally warm. Be sure to hydrate and listen to your body as well. (Jeff Galloway offers great tips as well, read the Official Event Guide or check out his website for more information.)

What are some tips to saving money during race weekends?
For accommodations, work with an Authorized Disney Vacation Planner. They will make sure that you are getting the best deal for your Walt Disney World Resort hotel or package. You can also room with friends and family to help cut down on cost. (Be sure to abide by the maximum number of guests in each room.) To cut down on food costs, you can also bring your own food along or eat off-property.

When does registration open for each runDisney race?
In Section E of the Appendix we have included all upcoming race registration dates for 2015 and into 2016.

Why can't I transfer my bib?
runDisney's policy states that bibs are non-transferrable and non-refundable. This is primarily due to safety and liability reasons. If anyone is to transfer their bib, the original runner and transferee are subject to disqualification.

More answers to Frequently Asked Questions can be found on runDisney.com.

B. Packing Lists

Sign up for the Magical Miles email list
(**http://bit.ly/MagicalMilesList**) to get a printable version.

1. Vacation
- Travel Documents (reservation numbers, passports, IDs)
- Shoes (multiple pair of tennis shoes, sandals)
- Shorts
- T-Shirts
- Sweatshirt/Jacket
- Jeans
- Swimsuit, Cover-up
- Hat, Sunglasses
- Backpack/Purse
- Camera, Charger, Memory Card
- Phone, Charger
- Toiletries (shampoo, soap, hair products, lotion)
- Toothbrush, Toothpaste
- Sunscreen, Aloe, Bug Spray
- Pain Medication (and other medication)
- Epsom Salts
- Band-Aids
- Rain Poncho, Umbrella
- Trash Bags, Ziploc Bags

2. Race Bag
- Race Waiver
- Shoes
- Clothes (race outfit)
- Socks
- Hat/Visor
- Garmin/GPS Watch
- iPod/mp3 Player
- Headphones
- Camera
- Phone
- Running belt
- Hydration belt/handheld

- Fuel (gels, sport beans, etc.)
- Body Glide
- Band-Aids
- Road ID
- Pre-Race Food
- Duct Tape
- Poncho or Trash Bag

3. **Bag Check**
- Wipes
- Towel
- Sweatshirt/Coat
- Flip-Flops/Sandals
- Resort Key
- ID
- Camera (if you don't run with it)
- Phone (if you don't run with it)
- Brush
- Mirror
- Chapstick
- Advil
- Gum
- Extra Clothes (night race)
- Extra Socks (night race)
- Tissues
- Food

C. Checklists for Expo and Before Race (in no particular order)

- Pick up race bib (and safety pins)
- Pick up race pins or commemorative items (if ordered)
- Shop for official race merchandise
- Enjoy speaker series
- Make support signs at Inspiration Station
- Get a pre-race massage, if needed
- Shop for race items
- Take pictures at different photo opportunity locations

D. Course Maps

Note: 2016 maps were not available at time of publication.

To see larger versions of the course maps, please visit
RunnersGuideToWDW.com/course-maps/.

Course Maps ©*Disney*

Walt Disney World 5K & 10K (January)

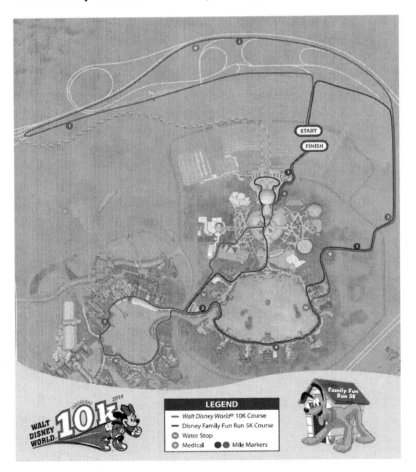

Walt Disney World Half-Marathon

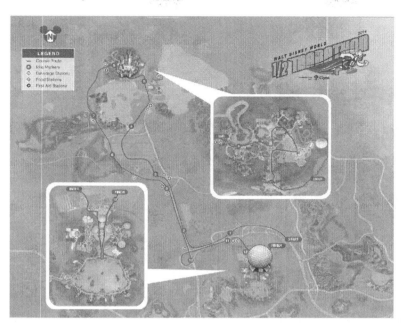

Walt Disney World Marathon

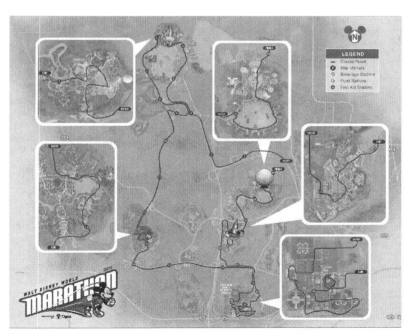

Star Wars 5K (Disneyland)

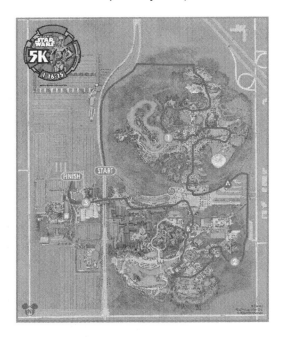

Star Wars 10K (Disneyland)

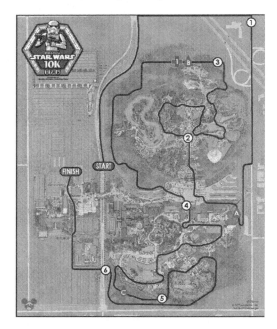

Star Wars Half-Marathon (Disneyland)

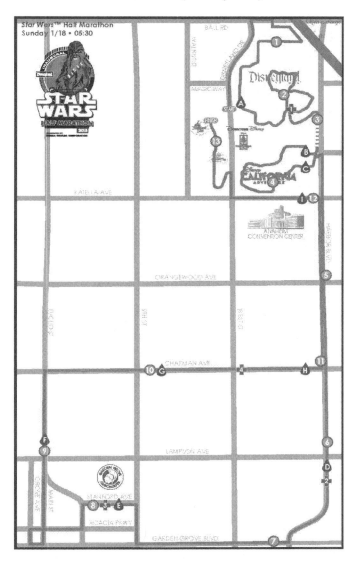

Princess 5K & 10K

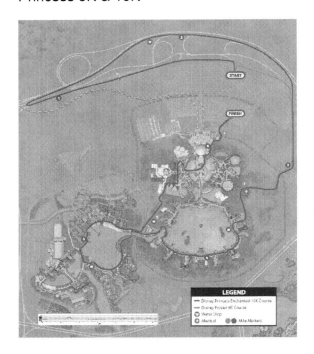

Princess Half-Marathon

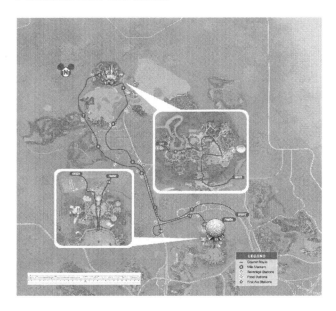

Neverland 5K

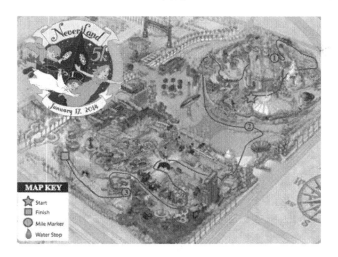

Tinker Bell 10K

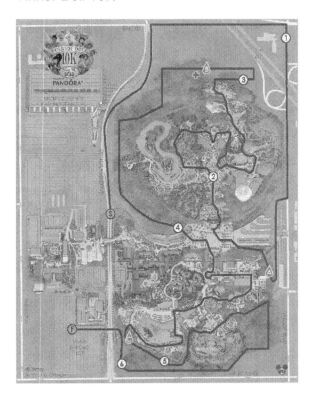

Tinker Bell Half-Marathon

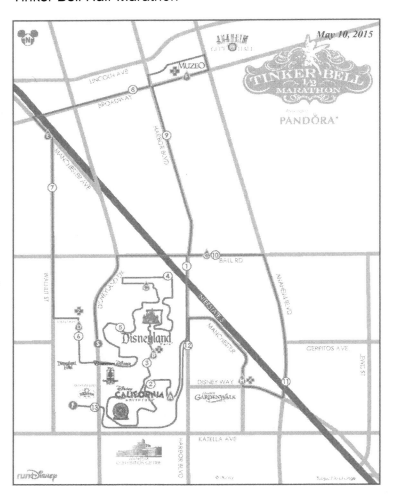

Disneyland 5K

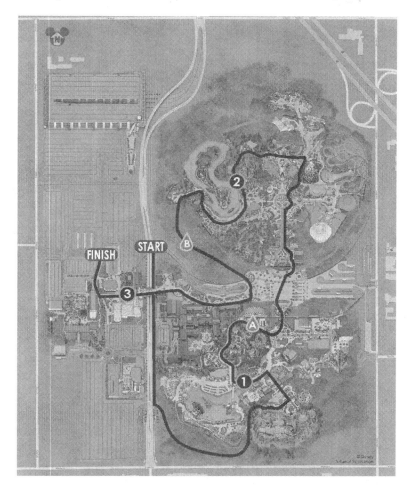

Disneyland 10K

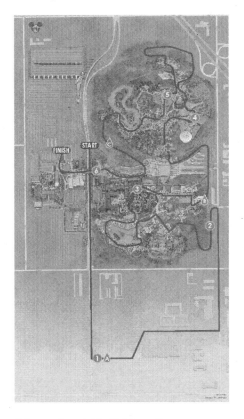

Disneyland Half-Marathon

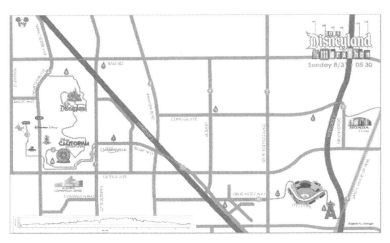

Mickey's Jingle Jungle 5K

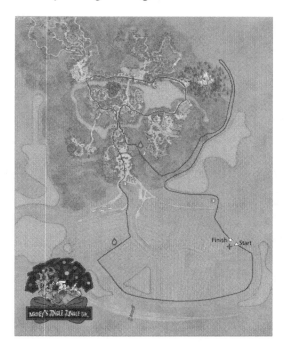

Wine & Dine Half-Marathon

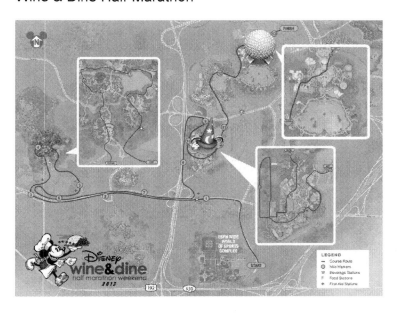

Avengers Super Heroes 5K

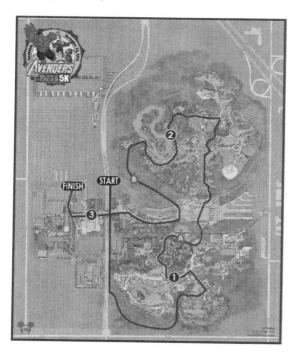

Avengers Super Heroes Half-Marathon

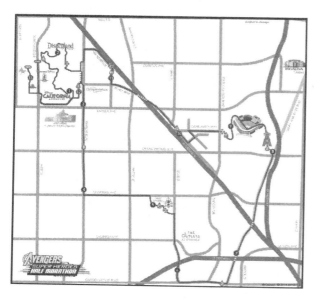

E. **Race Info**
Note: Race dates and times are subject to change. Please check **runDisney.com** for up-to-date information.

Walt Disney World Marathon Weekend

Dates: January 6-10, 2016 and January 4-8, 2017

Location: Walt Disney World Resort

Races Offered: Kids' Races, Mickey Mile, 5K, 10K, Half-Marathon, Marathon, Goofy's Race & A Half Challenge, Dopey Challenge

Race Info:
5K – January 7, 2016 – 6:00 a.m. – Start/Finish in Epcot
10K – January 8, 2016 – 5:30 a.m. – Start/Finish in Epcot
Half-Marathon – January 9, 2016 – 5:30 a.m – Start/Finish in Epcot
Marathon – January 10, 2016 – 5:30 a.m. – Start/Finish in Epcot

2016 Host Resorts: All on Walt Disney World property

2017 Registration Opens: April 26, 2016

Inaugural Event: 1998 – Half-Marathon, 1994 - Marathon, 2006 - Goofy's Race & a Half Challenge, 2014 – 10K and Dopey Challenge

Star Wars Half-Marathon Weekend

Dates: January 14-17, 2016 and January 12-15, 2017

Location: Disneyland Resort

Races Offered: Kids' Races, 5K, 10K, Half-Marathon, Rebel Challenge

Race Info:
5K – January 15, 2016 – 5:30 a.m. – Start/Finish at Disneyland Resort
10K – January 16, 2016 – 5:30 a.m. – Start/Finish at Disneyland Resort
Half-Marathon – January 17, 2016 – 5:30 a.m. – Start/Finish at Disneyland Resort

2017 Registration Opens: June 14, 2016

Inaugural Event: 2015 – 10K, Half-Marathon and Rebel Challenge

Princess Half-Marathon Weekend

Dates: February 18-21, 2016 and February 23-26, 2017

Location: Walt Disney World Resort

Races Offered: Kids' Races, 5K, 10K, Half-Marathon, Glass Slipper Challenge

Race Info:
5K – February 19, 2016 – 6:15 a.m. – Start/Finish in Epcot
10K – February 20, 2016 – 5:30 a.m. – Start/Finish in Epcot
Half-Marathon – February 21, 2016 – 5:30 a.m. – Start/Finish in Epcot

2016 Host Resorts: All on Walt Disney World property

2017 Registration Opens: July 12, 2016

Inaugural Event: 2009 – Half-Marathon, 2014 – 10K and Glass Slipper Challenge

Star Wars Half-Marathon Weekend – The Dark Side

Dates: April 14-17, 2016 and April 20-23, 2017

Location: Walt Disney Resort

Races Offered: Kids' Races, 5K, 10K, Half-Marathon, Dark Side Challenge

Race Info:
5K – April 15, 2016 – 6:00 a.m. – Start/Finish at Epcot
10K – April 16, 2016 – 5:30 a.m. – Start at Epcot, Finish at ESPN Wide World of Sports Complex

Half-Marathon – April 16, 2016 – 5:30 a.m. – Start at Epcot, Finish at ESPN Wide World of Sports Complex

2016 Host Resorts: TBD

2017 Registration Opens: August 9, 2016

Inaugural Event: 2016 – 10K, Half-Marathon and Dark Side Challenge

Tinker Bell Half-Marathon Weekend

Dates: May 5-8, 2016 and May 11-14, 2017

Location: Disneyland Resort

Races Offered: Kids' Races, 5K, 10K, Half-Marathon, Pixie Dust Challenge

Race Info:
5K – May 6, 2016 – 5:00 a.m. – Start/Finish at Disneyland Resort
10K – May 7, 2017 – 5:30 a.m. – Start/Finish at Disneyland Resort
Half-Marathon – May 8, 2016 – 5:30 a.m. – Start/Finish at Disneyland Resort

2017 Registration Opens: September 20, 2016

Inaugural Event: 2012 – Half-Marathon, 2014 – 10K, 2015 – Pixie Dust Challenge

Disneyland Half-Marathon Weekend

Dates: September 1-4, 2016

Location: Disneyland Resort

Races Offered: Kids' Races, 5K, 10K, Half-Marathon, Dumbo Double Dare

Race Info:

5K – September 4, 2015 – 5:30 a.m. – Start/Finish at Disneyland Resort
10K – September 5, 2015 – 6:15 a.m. - Start/Finish at Disneyland Resort
Half-Marathon – September 6, 2015 – 5:45 a.m. – Start/Finish at Disneyland Resort

2016 Registration Opens: February 2, 2016

Inaugural Event: 2006 – Half-Marathon, 2013 – 10K and Dumbo Double Dare

Wine & Dine Half-Marathon Weekend

Dates: November 6-7, 2015

Location: Walt Disney World Resort

Races Offered: Kids' Races, 5K, Half-Marathon

Race Info:
5K – November 7, 2015 – 7:00 a.m. – Start/Finish in Animal Kingdom
Half-Marathon – November 7, 2015 – 10:00 p.m. – Start at ESPN Wide World of Sports, Finish in Epcot

2015 Host Resorts: Disney's All-Star Resorts, Disney's Pop Century, Disney's Caribbean Beach Resort, Disney's Port Orleans-Riverside Resort, Disney's Port Orleans-French Quarter Resort, Disney's Saratoga Springs Resort & Spa, Disney's Beach Club Resort, Disney's Boardwalk Inn, Disney's Polynesian Resort, Disney's Wilderness Lodge and Disney's Yacht Club Resort. *(2016 Host Resorts not available at time of publication.)*

2016 Registration Opens: March 15, 2016

Inaugural Event: 2010

Avengers Super Heroes Half-Marathon Weekend

Dates: November 12-15, 2015

Location: Disneyland Resort

Races Offered: Kids' Races, 5K, Half-Marathon

Race Info:
5K – November 14, 2015 – 5:30 a.m. – Start/Finish at Disneyland Resort
Half-Marathon – November 15, 2015 – 5:30 a.m. – Start/Finish at Disneyland Resort

2016 Registration Opens: April 5, 2016

Inaugural Event: 2014 – Half-Marathon, 2015 – Captain America 10K and Infinity Gauntlet Challenge

Connect

Email - info@runnersguidetoWDW.com

Website/Blog - RunnersGuideToWDW.com

Twitter - twitter.com/RunWDW

Facebook - facebook.com/RunnersGuideToWDW

Instagram - instagram.com/RunWDW

Pinterest - pinterest.com/RunWDW

About the Authors

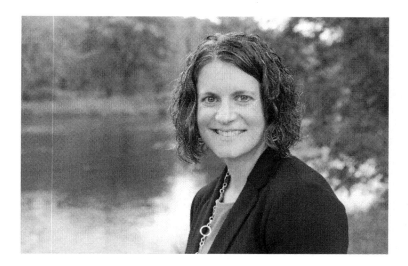

Megan Biller is an avid runner and Disney enthusiast and has been visiting Walt Disney World since she was just a toddler. The love of Disney only grew as she continued to visit the parks and sail on the cruise line. Having been athletic all her life, she took to running, and has experienced multiple runDisney events – falling in love with each and every one. Her husband is a recurrent ChEAR Squad member and personal photographer for her events, encouraging her along the way. As a gluten free runner, Megan has insight on the best gluten free meals at Walt Disney World.

Megan is currently training for the Walt Disney World Marathon in January 2016 as well as the inaugural Disneyland Paris Half-Marathon. Megan lives in Michigan with her husband.

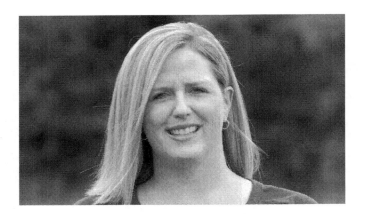

Krista Albrecht is an avid recreational runner who has completed numerous 10Ks, runDisney events and the New York City Marathon. She visits various Disney destinations multiple times each year with her family. From the Kids' Races to the Goofy Race and a Half Challenge, all members of her family have participated in runDisney races. Along with participating in runDisney events, she has also served as cheerleader for her husband who has completed the Goofy Race and Half Challenge twice and her daughter who is an avid competitor in the 200m Dash at Disney's Kids' Race.

Krista will be back again for the Glass Slipper Challenge in February 2016 along with the inaugural Star Wars Half-Marathon Weekend – The Dark Side. Krista currently resides in Florida with her husband and daughter.

Index